STUDY GUID

Medical Assisting Made

Incredibly
Easy

LAB
COMPETENCIES

STUDY GUIDE FOR

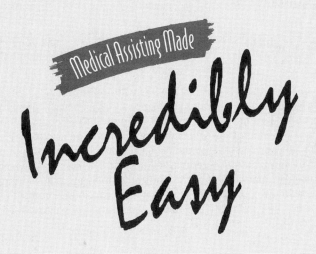

LAB
COMPETENCIES

Peter J. Doolin, MT (ASCP), MEd, RMA

Medical Department
McFatter Technical Center
Davie, Florida

Wolters Kluwer | Lippincott Williams & Wilkins
Health
Philadelphia · Baltimore · New York · London
Buenos Aires · Hong Kong · Sydney · Tokyo

Executive Editor: John Goucher
Senior Managing Editor: Rebecca Kerins
Marketing Manager: Hilary Henderson
Production Manager: Eve Malakoff-Klein
Illustrator: Bot Roda
Designer: Joan Wendt
Compositor: Circle Graphics, Inc.
Printer: Victor Graphics, Inc.

9 8 7 6 5 4 3 2

DISCLAIMER

Care has been taken to confirm the accuracy of the information present and to describe generally accepted practices. However, the authors, editors, and publisher are not responsible for errors or omissions or for any consequences from application of the information in this book and make no warranty, expressed or implied, with respect to the currency, completeness, or accuracy of the contents of the publication. Application of this information in a particular situation remains the professional responsibility of the practitioner; the clinical treatments described and recommended may not be considered absolute and universal recommendations.

The authors, editors, and publisher have exerted every effort to ensure that drug selection and dosage set forth in this text are in accordance with the current recommendations and practice at the time of publication. However, in view of ongoing research, changes in government regulations, and the constant flow of information relating to drug therapy and drug reactions, the reader is urged to check the package insert for each drug for any change in indications and dosage and for added warnings and precautions. This is particularly important when the recommended agent is a new or infrequently employed drug.

Some drugs and medical devices presented in this publication have Food and Drug Administration (FDA) clearance for limited use in restricted research settings. It is the responsibility of the health care provider to ascertain the FDA status of each drug or device planned for use in their clinical practice.

To purchase additional copies of this book, call our customer service department at **(800) 638-3030** or fax orders to **(301) 223-2320**. International customers should call **(301) 223-2300**.

Visit Lippincott Williams & Wilkins on the Internet: http://www.lww.com. Lippincott Williams & Wilkins customer service representatives are available from 8:30 am to 6:00 p.m., EST.

PREFACE

Welcome to the *Study Guide for Medical Assisting Made Incredibly Easy: Lab Competencies!* The activities and exercises in this book will help you retain important information, master skills, and become a success as a medical assistant. To help you get the most out of your studies, we've included a variety of exercises that will help reinforce the material you learned and build your critical thinking skills. As you work through the book, take note of the helpful study tips presented by Maria, a Certified Medical Assistant, who guides you through the material.

Special Features

Learning Objectives serve as a guide as you review your text. You'll be expected to master each learning and performance objective.

Learning Self-Assessment Exercises include crossword puzzles, procedure practice exercises, labeling exercises, word searches, word scrambles, critical thinking practice exercises, and practice quizzes. Your instructor has the answer key to these exercises.

Certification Prep includes questions that will help you prepare for the Medical Assisting Certification Examination. Your instructor has the answers to these questions, too.

Competency Evaluation Forms

The competency evaluation forms included at the end of chapters 2–7 are designed to help you practice and test your proficiency in many of the skills you'll be responsible for knowing as a medical assistant. At the beginning of the book, a Competency Evaluation Tracking Form is included so you can record in one place where and when each procedure was completed. On each competency evaluation form, you'll find a Hands On procedure broken down step-by-step and a list of equipment and materials you'll need to do the procedure. Before you start, your instructor will tell you how long you'll have to complete the procedure and what the passing score will be.

HOW TO CALCULATE YOUR SCORE

Each form has three columns. The first column is for self-evaluation, the second is for your partner's evaluation, and the third is for your instructor's evaluation. You'll find that having two chances to practice the skills on your own will help you remember the information. It will also build your confidence for when you have to complete the procedure for your instructor during a test.

You can earn one of three possible scores for each step in the procedure:

4 = satisfactory

0 = unsatisfactory

NA = not counted

Each procedure has a total number of points that can be earned. To get this number, add the number of steps and multiply that number by 4. To calculate your score, add the number of points you earned and multiply that number by 100. Divide this number by the total possible points, and you'll get your final percentage.

Together with its accompanying main text, this *Study Guide for Medical Assisting Made Incredibly Easy: Lab Competencies* is designed to make the study of medical assisting fun and effective. The purpose of this book, and the entire *Medical Assisting Made Incredibly Easy* series, is student success!

CONTENTS

Competency Evaluation Tracking Form

Student Name _____

Hands On Procedure	Page No.	School Class/Lab Date/Initials	Externship Site #1 Date/Initials	Externship Site #2 Date/Initials	Externship Site #3 Date/Initials
2-1 Obtaining a Blood Specimen by Venipuncture	19				
2-2 Obtaining a Blood Specimen by Skin Puncture	23				
3-1 Preparing a Whole Blood Dilution Using the Unopette System	35				
3-2 Making a Peripheral Blood Smear	37				
3-3 Staining a Peripheral Blood Smear	39				
3-4 Performing a White Blood Cell Differential	41				
3-5 Performing a Manual Microhematocrit Determination	43				
3-6 Performing a Westergren Erythrocyte Sedimentation Rate	45				
4-1 Performing an HCG Pregnancy Test	57				
4-2 Performing a Group A Rapid Strep Test	59				
5-1 Obtaining a Clean-Catch Midstream Urine Specimen	71				
5-2 Performing a Chemical Strip Analysis	75				
5-3 Determining the Color and Clarity of Urine	79				
5-4 Performing a Clinitest for Reducing Sugars	81				
5-5 Performing a Nitroprusside Reaction (ACETEST) for Ketones	85				
5-6 Performing an Acid Precipitation Test for Protein	87				

Competency Evaluation Tracking Form (continued)

Student Name _____

Hands On Procedure	Page No.	School Class/Lab Date/Initials	Externship Site #1 Date/Initials	Externship Site #2 Date/Initials	Externship Site #3 Date/Initials
5-7 Performing the Diazo Tablet Test (Ictotest) for Bilirubin	91				
5-8 Preparing Urine Sediment	93				
6-1 Determining Blood Glucose	103				
6-2 Glucose Tolerance Testing	105				
7-1 Collecting a Specimen for Throat Culture	117				
7-2 Collecting a Sputum Specimen	119				
7-3 Collecting a Stool Specimen	121				
7-4 Testing a Stool Specimen for Occult Blood	123				
7-5 Inoculating a Culture Using Dilution Streaking	125				
7-6 Inoculating for Drug Sensitivity Testing (Kirby-Bauer Disk Diffusion Drug Sensitivity) Using "Even Lawn" Streaking	127				
7-7 Inoculating for Quantitative Culturing or Urine Colony Count Using "Even Lawn" Streaking	131				
7-8 Preparing a Wet Mount Slide	135				
7-9 Preparing a Dry Smear	137				
7-10 Gram Staining a Smear Slide	141				
7-11 Performing Wound Collection Procedure for Microbiological Testing	145				

Chapter 1

GETTING TO KNOW THE CLINICAL LAB

Chapter Competencies

Review the information in your textbook that supports the
following course objectives.

It's important to know and understand proper lab safety procedures not just to pass the test and do well in class, but also to protect yourself and your coworkers while working in a lab.

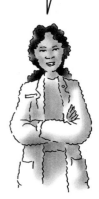

Learning Objectives

- List the reasons for lab tests
- Describe the medical assistant's role in the lab
- Identify the kinds of labs where medical assistants work and describe what these labs do
- List the kinds of people who work in a lab and the duties of each
- Name each type of lab department and explain what it does
- List the equipment found in most small labs and explain its purpose
- Identify the kinds of hazards encountered in a lab and summarize how to deal with them
- Explain how OSHA makes labs safer
- List the safe behaviors employees should practice in the lab
- Identify CLIA and explain how it affects lab operations
- Describe how quality control affects lab operations

Learning Self-Assessment Exercises

KEY TERMS

Complete the crossword puzzle below with the appropriate key terms.

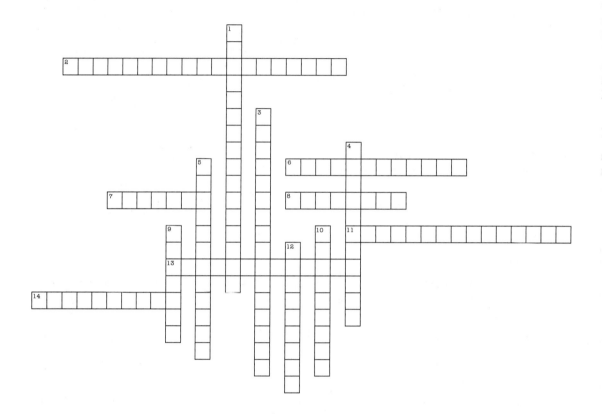

ACROSS

2. dangerous organisms that can exist in the blood of an infected person
6. acceptable ranges for healthy people that lab results are compared to
7. particles suspended in gas or air
8. a body sample like stool, blood, or urine
11. the range of tests an analyzer, instrument, or procedure is capable of producing results for
13. anything that prevents or delays the clotting of blood
14. a machine that separates liquids into different parts

DOWN

1. an evaluation of health care services as compared to accepted standards
3. a spinning motion to exert force outward with heavier components spinning downward
4. setting the calculation points for the instrument by processing solutions of known values within the reportable range of the instrument
5. a person who draws blood from a patient
9. chemical used to produce a test reaction
10. something that is marked at intervals (as in a container) in order to allow the measurement of its contents
12. the middle layer of a blood specimen containing white blood cells and platelets that forms when blood has been centrifuged

> If you're having trouble memorizing key terms or ideas, try creating flash cards. Then you can quiz yourself and practice those terms that give you a hard time.

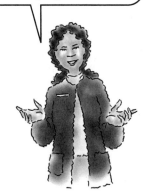

PROCEDURE PRACTICE

Following Chain of Custody

Below is a sequence chart for following the chain of custody (COC) when collecting specimens for drug testing. Fill in the missing steps with the choices from the answer bank on the next page.

1. Obtain a picture ID and have the subject empty his pockets before collecting the specimen.

↓

2. _____

_____

↓

3. Record whether or not collection of the specimen was witnessed.

↓

4. _____

_____

↓

5. Have the subject and the collector sign the COC form, with the date and time of collection.

↓

6. _____

_____

↓

7. _____

_____

↓

8. _____

_____

ANSWER BANK

➤ Seal the bag for transport to the testing facility.

➤ Record the specimen's temperature (90.5°F to 99.8°F is acceptable). Its minimum volume should be 35 mL.

➤ The water supply in the restroom used for collection must be turned off. A dye must be added to the toilet water to prevent the subject from using it as the specimen.

➤ Put the specimen and COC form in a tamper-proof bag.

➤ Sign and attach tamper seals to each side of the container.

LABELING

Let's see how well you know the microscope. Look at the picture on the next page and fill in the names for each labeled part.

1. _____

2. _____

3. _____

4. _____

5. _____

6. _____

7. _____

8. _____

9. _____

10. _____

11. _____

12. _____

PRACTICE QUIZ

1. Lab testing is done for all of the following reasons except:
   a. to cure a disease.
   b. to determine an individual's normal values.
   c. to diagnose a disease.
   d. to determine the progress of a disease.

2. Which of the following is NOT commonly performed in a physician office lab (POL)?
   a. cholesterol levels
   b. hematocrit
   c. stool analysis
   d. urinalysis

3. Which of the following steps is NOT necessary for proper care of a microscope?
   a. Keep the microscope away from any vibrating equipment.
   b. Make sure the light source is turned off when storing the microscope.
   c. Clean the ocular lens with a piece of gauze after each use.
   d. Always carry the microscope with one hand on the base and one on the arm.

4. The clinical chemistry department of a POL does which of the following?
   a. tests for diseases
   b. tests for drugs in the blood
   c. tests for cancer in surgically removed tissues
   d. tests for the number of white blood cells in the blood

5. In a centrifuged blood sample, platelets would be found in what layer?
   a. surface
   b. top layer
   c. middle layer
   d. bottom layer

Although you can consult manuals while you're working in the lab, you'll be a step ahead if you memorize the parts and pieces of various lab equipment.

6. What is a function of an immunohematology department?
   a. perform blood typing on donor blood
   b. research microbes that might be harmful to blood
   c. study the reproduction rate of bacteria in blood
   d. analyze the levels of hormones in blood

7. Which of the following statements about using a centrifuge is NOT true?
   a. An unbalanced centrifuge could fall off the table.
   b. Never stop the centrifuge spinning with your hand.
   c. There must be an even number of tubes in the centrifuge.
   d. The centrifuge tubes should not be capped.

8. Why is it important to follow the chain of custody when obtaining a specimen for drug testing?
   a. It is easier to track the different labs the specimen travels to.
   b. It ensures the specimen is legitimate.
   c. It prevents two different people's specimens from being mixed up.
   d. It shows that the person followed the right procedures when preparing to give the specimen.

9. Which piece of equipment is correctly paired with its job?
   a. Graduated cylinder: container used for measuring liquids
   b. Flask: container with a wide opening for mixing or heating liquids
   c. Test tube: container with a narrow opening and round base for holding or moving liquids
   d. Beaker: straw-shaped container open on one end and rounded on the other end; it holds lab specimens

10. The study of fungi is called:
    a. bacteriology.
    b. virology.
    c. mycology.
    d. parasitology.

CRITICAL THINKING PRACTICE

Lab Safety

Below are scenarios that you witness in the lab. Explain if the worker is following proper lab procedure and what he or she can do to promote lab safety.

1. Marcus doesn't have time for lunch because he has so many lab tests to run during the day. He brings his bottled water and an apple into the lab for a quick snack before he can stop for a real lunch.

_____

_____

2. Sherry has been working in the lab all morning centrifuging blood samples. When she finishes that job, she reviews some new MSDS for new chemicals the lab is working with. While she reviews the paperwork, she chews on the top of her pen cap.

_____

_____

3. Mustafa washes his hands and enters the lab. Before he can start to work, he receives a page that he has a phone call. He washes his hands and leaves the lab. When he returns, he washes his hands and then reviews his charts to see what work he has to get done.

_____

_____

4. Lin is removing the stopper from a container filled with a specimen. While doing this, she holds the mouth of the container away from herself and her lab partner.

_____

_____

5. Alicia has to leave work at 5:00 P.M. for an appointment. She looks at the clock and realizes she has only five minutes. She removes her gloves and washes her hands. Then she makes a note that she will disinfect the lab surfaces first thing in the morning because she is running late.

> Lab safety is essential to your career as a medical assistant. To practice good habits, try role playing various scenes in a lab with a partner.

_____

_____

Occupational Safety and Health Administration Requirements

There are two important Occupational Safety and Health Administration (OSHA) standards that apply to medical labs:

- The Occupational Exposure to Bloodborne Pathogens Standard
- The Hazardous Communication (HazCom) Standard

Read the statements below and identify which standard is being discussed. Explain your answer.

1. You trip while carrying a specimen cup and the collected body fluid splashes up in your eyes and nose. Which OSHA standard applies to this situation? Why?

_____

_____

_____

2. You're working with a new chemical in the lab and you're unclear if the material is dangerous or flammable. You look for the label on the product to answer your question. Which OSHA standard applies to this situation? Why?

_____

_____

_____

3. You start working at a new lab. Your boss schedules you for free immunization against hepatitis B virus. Which OSHA standard applies to this situation? Why?

_____

_____

_____

4. You're conducting tests using a centrifuge and your supervisor says you must wear a face shield and shoe covers in addition to the disposable gloves you normally wear. Which OSHA standard applies to this situation? Why?

_____

_____

_____

5. Your supervisor asks you to store a chemical that you just used in the lab. She says you must consult the MSDS before you put the substance away. Which OSHA standard applies to this situation? Why?

_____

_____

_____

Certification Prep

1. The generic term for a disease-causing microbe that lives and transmits through blood is:
   a. aerobic pathogen.
   b. hemolytic bacteria.
   c. bloodborne pathogen.
   d. anaerobic pathogen.

2. Plasma is:
   a. the hemoglobin.
   b. the fibrinogen.
   c. the liquid portion of the blood containing white blood cells that makes up 75% of whole blood.
   d. the clear liquid portion of the blood comprising 55% of whole blood.

3. Which of the following is a chemical agent used to clean counter tops and exam tables?
   a. disinfectant
   b. antibiotic
   c. antiseptic
   d. sterile solution

4. The clear portion of the blood after clotting and centrifuging is:
   a. plasma.
   b. serum.
   c. buffy coat.
   d. hemoglobin.

5. Which department of the laboratory performs tests to determine if antibodies against a particular disease are present?
   a. immunology
   b. chemistry
   c. microbiology
   d. histology

6. What is the study of histology?
   a. the microscopic study of bacteria
   b. the microscopic study of antigens
   c. the microscopic study of antibodies
   d. the microscopic study of tissues

7. In which lab department are specimens planted and grown in appropriate media?
   a. microbiology
   b. immunology
   c. hematology
   d. chemistry

8. What is pathology?
   a. the study of microscopic mutations
   b. the study of the cause and effect of disease
   c. the study of cell division and reproduction
   d. the study of transference

9. What federal agency monitors and protects the health and safety of workers?
   a. U.S. Department of Labor
   b. Occupational Safety and Health Administration
   c. National Bureau of Labor
   d. National Bureau of Occupational Safety

10. What is a reagent?
   a. a set of standards by which a laboratory calibrates equipment
   b. a control sample, with a known result, that is tested in conjunction with a patient sample
   c. a district representative of CLIA, who performs surprise laboratory inspections
   d. a chemical used to produce a reaction in a testing situation

Chapter 2

PHLEBOTOMY

Chapter Competencies

Review the information in your textbook that supports the following course objectives.

> Don't skip breakfast in the morning. This meal will give you the energy you need during your classes and study time.

Learning Objectives

- Identify the main methods of phlebotomy
- Identify equipment and supplies used in routine venipuncture and skin puncture.
- List the major additives, their color codes, and the suggested order in which they are filled from a venipuncture
- Perform venipuncture and describe proper site selection and needle positioning
- Perform skin puncture
- Identify complications of venipuncture and skin puncture and how to prevent them
- Explain how to handle exposure to bloodborne pathogens

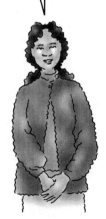

Learning Self-Assessment Exercises

KEY TERMS

Complete the word search puzzle on the next page with the appropriate key terms. Words may be backwards and diagonal, and letters may be used for more than one clue. (Hint: It may be helpful to determine which words you are seeking before searching the puzzle.)

```
S  C  Y  W  W  Y  B  M  W  V  B  V  R  V  V  Y  C  A
Y  H  E  M  O  L  Y  S  I  S  E  L  A  U  R  B  I  N
N  H  M  O  O  S  T  V  J  N  B  C  E  A  R  O  T  T
C  D  H  B  T  T  G  R  I  N  U  Q  L  V  T  U  P  E
O  E  G  U  A  G  O  P  L  U  P  L  E  Y  E  A  E  C
P  W  N  P  G  N  U  B  M  L  I  G  C  Y  Q  B  S  U
E  P  R  T  C  N  B  B  E  P  S  C  K  C  J  C  I  B
W  P  H  A  C  S  I  X  A  L  Y  H  P  O  R  P  T  I
D  U  D  T  W  Z  R  C  O  H  H  H  T  I  S  U  N  T
R  S  U  R  X  Q  F  I  S  Y  E  P  F  N  Q  Y  A  A
D  R  G  K  Y  I  I  K  L  R  F  M  D  M  E  B  Y  L
E  O  U  Z  C  K  P  V  A  G  E  V  A  X  H  J  S  S
H  E  M  O  C  O  N  C  E  N  T  R  A  T  I  O  N  P
H  I  Y  C  F  V  Y  Y  L  A  Y  N  A  J  O  U  M  A
Z  J  K  A  K  J  Z  Q  P  W  K  W  T  Y  T  M  L  C
Q  Y  H  M  N  J  S  F  R  H  I  S  P  N  T  Z  A  E
Z  P  Z  L  T  M  G  E  C  X  Q  C  G  W  Q  V  E  E
A  C  K  N  Z  I  P  R  P  J  V  X  K  U  L  R  H  X
```

1. the process of collecting blood
2. the size of the opening in a needle
3. the pooling of blood components
4. a very small blood vessel
5. the slanted cut at the end of a needle that allows a needle to penetrate a vein easily
6. a hollow needle used to puncture a vein
7. fainting or loss of consciousness
8. the rupturing of blood cells
9. inner surface of the bend of the elbow where the major veins for venipuncture are located
10. a space from which air has been removed
11. this forms when blood leaks into the tissues during a venipuncture procedure
12. a substance that can block the growth of bacteria
13. protective treatment for the prevention of disease once exposure has occurred

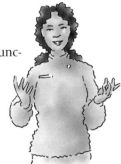

Caffeine is fine in small doses, but it's not a good idea to drink an entire pot of coffee at night in order to stay up and study.

PROCEDURE PRACTICE

Obtaining Blood Specimens by Skin Puncture

Below is a sequence chart for performing a skin puncture to obtain a blood specimen. Fill in the missing steps with the choices from the answer bank on pages 13 and 14.

1. Check the requisition slip to see what tests have been ordered. Also note the specimen requirements.

↓

2. _____

_____

↓

3. Wash your hands.

↓

4. _____

_____

↓

5. Put on gloves. Follow standard precautions.

↓

6. _____

_____

↓

7. _____

_____

↓

8. You'll use both hands for this procedure. Grasp the finger or heel firmly with your nondominant hand. Now clean the area with alcohol and wipe dry.

↓

9. While you hold the finger or heel firmly, make a swift, firm puncture using your dominant hand.
   - After puncture, the dispose of the used puncture device in a sharps container.
   - Wipe away the first drop of blood. It may be contaminated with tissue fluid or residue from your alcohol wipe.
   - Apply pressure toward the site.

10. _____

    _____

11. _____

    _____

12. Thank your patient when you've finished. Tell your patient to leave the bandage in place for at least 30 minutes.

13. _____

    _____

14. _____

    _____

ANSWER BANK

➤ Select the puncture site. It will be one of the following:
   (A) just off center of the tip of the middle or ring finger of the nondominant hand
   (B) the lateral curved surface of the heel
   (C) the heel of an infant

➤ Once you've collected the blood you need, apply clean gauze to the site with pressure or have the patient apply pressure. Don't release your patient until the bleeding has stopped. Label the containers with the proper information.

➤ Assemble your equipment.

➤ Make sure the site you've chosen is warm. Gently massage the finger from the base to the tip to increase blood flow.

(*continued on next page*)

➤ Test, transfer, or store the specimen according to your office's policy, and record the procedure.

➤ To finish your task, take care of or dispose of equipment and supplies. Clean your work area. Then you can remove your gloves and wash your hands.

➤ Greet and identify the patient. Explain the procedure and answer any questions.

➤ Collect the specimen. You can encourage blood flow by holding the puncture site downward and applying gentle pressure near the site.

Methods of Blood Collection

There are two main methods used to collect blood—venipuncture and skin puncture. For each of the statements below, write in V if it applies to venipuncture and SP if it applies to skin puncture.

Try to get eight hours of sleep at night so you feel rested when you wake up.

_____ 1. The type of blood vessel used is a vein.

_____ 2. The type of blood vessel used is a capillary.

_____ 3. Evacuated tubes are used to collect blood.

_____ 4. A lancet is used to collect blood.

_____ 5. Microcollection containers are used to collect blood.

_____ 6. Microhematocrit tubes are used to collect blood.

_____ 7. A needle and tourniquet are used to collect blood.

_____ 8. This method is used when only a few drops of blood are needed.

_____ 9. A tourniquet may be applied to assist with the procedure.

_____ 10. This method is commonly used for point-of-care testing outside of the lab.

PRACTICE QUIZ

1. Which of the following is NOT equipment needed by a phlebotomist?
   a. antibiotic
   b. antiseptic
   c. gauze
   d. gloves

2. Which of the following statements about the evacuated tube system is true?
   a. Which colored stopper to use is determined by which blood test is being conducted.
   b. You should remove the same amount of blood from every patient so there is enough for testing.
   c. Additives should never be added to the evacuated tube system because they make the blood go bad.
   d. It is best to use the same colored stopper for all the tests a patient needs so they don't get confused with another patient's tubes.

3. Why is it helpful to palpate a vein before drawing blood?
   a. Palpating helps the blood to clot.
   b. Palpating helps the blood move faster through the veins.
   c. Palpating helps to determine the size, depth, and direction of a vein.
   d. Palpating helps blood to divide into the different blood components.

4. The most common complication of venipuncture is:
   a. clotting.
   b. hematoma.
   c. irregular heartbeat.
   d. excessive blood loss.

5. Which of the following procedures should you follow when drawing blood from a patient who is prone to fainting?
   a. Give the patient a small snack or a drink before the procedure.
   b. Have the patient lie down during the procedure so she won't fall.
   c. Use two tourniquets to help the vein enlarge and fill with blood faster.
   d. Have a coworker hold the patient in his chair in case he starts to fall out.

6. Why do phlebotomists use tourniquets when collecting blood by venipuncture?
   a. It constricts the muscles in the arm to control blood flow.
   b. It enlarges the veins so they are easier to find and puncture.
   c. It slows down the blood flow in the veins so the person stops bleeding faster.
   d. It keeps the person's arm stable so the person is not injured during the blood collection.

7. Skin puncture can be used in all of the following situations except:
   a. when collecting blood from infants.
   b. when collecting blood from burn patients.
   c. when collecting large volumes of blood.
   d. when collecting small volumes of blood.

8. Which of the following instruments is NOT correctly paired with its method of blood collection?
   a. evacuated tubes—venipuncture
   b. syringe system—skin puncture
   c. winged infusion set—venipuncture
   d. microhematocrit tubes—skin puncture

9. Why would a phlebotomist use a warming device on an infant?
   a. Warmers make the veins pop out of the skin so it's easier to insert the needle.
   b. Warmers slow down the blood flow so it's easier to draw.
   c. Warmers help the blood to clot.
   d. Warmers increase blood flow before skin is punctured.

10. OSHA requires that all needles have a safety feature to prevent:
    a. needle stick injuries.
    b. the needle being used more than five times.
    c. the needle from being given to the wrong patient.
    d. the patient from administering the needle to him or herself.

CRITICAL THINKING PRACTICE

Sources of Errors in Phlebotomy

Consider the following situations involving venipuncture and skin puncture techniques. Did the medical assistant follow proper medical procedure or are there errors in the process? Mark each situation *Correct* or *Incorrect* and explain your answer, including suggestions on how you might have done things differently if any errors were made.

1. Rhonda asks the patient if she followed dietary restrictions and fasted before giving blood. The patient gets upset and says that she forgot. Rhonda says that's fine and continues with the procedure.

   Correct   Incorrect

   _____

   _____

2. Miguel starts by introducing himself to the patient and explaining the procedure. When he starts looking on the right arm for a vein, the patient suggests he tries the left arm instead because it is easier to find a vein there. Miguel takes this advice and finds a vein on the left arm.

   Correct   Incorrect

   _____

   _____

3. Rosa applies the tourniquet three inches above the site from which she plans to take blood on the left arm. Even with the tourniquet on, she can't find a good vein. She tells the patient that she will keep it on for two minutes and asks the patient to open and close his fist to help the process.

   Correct   Incorrect

   _____

   _____

4. Costas is busy drawing blood when the patient says he feels faint. Costas tells the patient to try to focus on something else because the procedure will be over in less than a minute. He encourages the patient to hang on and speaks patiently to him while he finishes drawing the blood.

   Correct   Incorrect

   _____

   _____

Choosing a Needle Gauge

1. You need to collect a blood sample from an infant. Which needle gauge would you use—a 20 or 23? Explain why.

   _____

   _____

2. Your patient has tortuous veins. Explain this condition, and then choose between a 21- or a 23-gauge needle.

   _____

   _____

3. When would you use a 24-gauge needle to collect blood?

   _____

   _____

Certification Prep

1. How does warming a venipuncture site improve the blood draw process?
   a. It causes the skin cells to relax and thin, making visualization of veins easier.
   b. It brings veins to the surface so the venipuncture isn't as deep.
   c. It increases blood flow, which causes veins to fill.
   d. It helps the patient to relax, which promotes vasodilation.

2. Which tube would you use to draw a sample for serum?
   a. red top
   b. purple top
   c. light blue top
   d. dark green top

3. You are to draw blood from an elderly person with small veins. What needle size will you use?
   a. 22 gauge
   b. 20 gauge
   c. 24 gauge
   d. 18 gauge

4. What is the reason for using a tourniquet or inflated blood pressure cuff during venipuncture?
   a. Either one may help hold the person's sleeve up out of the way.
   b. Either one will make the veins more prominent and easier to puncture.
   c. It distracts the patient by causing discomfort in an area other than the puncture site.
   d. The pressure on the vein will help the blood tubes to fill quickly.

5. What is the best way to confirm that you are drawing blood from the right patient?
    a. Ask the patient to say his name and compare it to the name on the order form.
    b. See if the person who responded to your call looks to be the age indicated on the form.
    c. Compare the patient name and account number with the computer database.
    d. Ask the nurse what the patient looks like.

6. What is a good question to ask a patient before performing a venipuncture?
    a. When was the last time you had blood drawn?
    b. I'm a student in training; would you prefer an experienced phlebotomist to do this?
    c. Would you mind if I don't wear gloves, since I can feel the vein better without them?
    d. Might this make you lightheaded? If so, would you like to lie down?

7. What are the main veins used for venipuncture?
    a. hepatic, renal, and cardiac
    b. brachial, carotid, and cephalic
    c. femoral, brachial, and renal
    d. cephalic, basilica, and median

8. What is an advantage of using butterfly needles?
    a. They work well for small veins and may be stabilized by taping in place.
    b. They are color coded, which makes them convenient to use when in a hurry.
    c. They are cost effective compared with other types of needles.
    d. They prompt a better flashback of blood to show that they are in the vein.

9. The red top blood collection tube:
    a. contains an anticoagulant.
    b. is empty.
    c. contains a preservative.
    d. contains a serum separating gel.

10. The medical term for fainting is:
    a. sepsis.
    b. shock.
    c. syncope.
    d. anaphylaxis.

Hands On ⚡ **Procedure 2-1:** Obtaining a Blood Specimen by Venipuncture

Task: With your partner as the patient, obtain a blood specimen by venipuncture.

Conditions: The student will perform this task under the conditions described in the Procedure Steps, below.

Equipment/Supplies: needle, syringe, test tubes, or evacuated tubes; tourniquet; sterile gauze pads; bandages; needle and adaptor; sharps container; 70-percent alcohol pad or other antiseptic; permanent marker or pen; biohazard barriers such as gloves, impervious gown, and face shield

Standards: The student will perform this skill with _____ % accuracy in a total of _____ minutes. *(Your instructor will tell you what the percentage and time limits will be before you begin.)*

Key: 4 = Satisfactory   0 = Unsatisfactory   NA = this step is not counted

Procedure Steps	Self	Partner	Instructor
1. Check the requisition slip to see what tests have been ordered. Also note the specimen requirements.	☐	☐	☐
2. Assemble your equipment. Don't use any equipment that has expired.	☐	☐	☐
3. Wash your hands.	☐	☐	☐
4. Greet and identify the patient. Explain the procedure and answer any questions. If the patient was required to fast, ask how long it's been since she ate. (It should have been at least eight hours.)	☐	☐	☐
5. Put on nonsterile latex gloves. Follow standard precautions.	☐	☐	☐
6. Get your needle ready by following procedures for using a syringe or an evacuated tube.	☐	☐	☐
7. Ask the patient to sit with a well-supported arm. Veins in the antecubital fossa are easiest to locate when the arm is straight to a 15-degree bend at the elbow.	☐	☐	☐

Continued on back

	Self	Partner	Instructor
8. Apply the tourniquet around the patient's arm three to four inches above the elbow. Check that it is snug but not too tight. Secure by using a half-bow knot. Make sure the tails of the tourniquet go toward the shoulder. Ask the patient to make a fist. Tell her to hold the fist and not to pump it.	☐	☐	☐
9. Using your gloved index finger, palpate to find a vein. Then trace the vein with your finger.	☐	☐	☐
10. Release the tourniquet.	☐	☐	☐
11. Cleanse the venipuncture site with an alcohol pad. Allow it to dry or dry with sterile gauze. Don't touch the site after cleansing.	☐	☐	☐
12. If you're drawing blood for a blood culture, be sure the specimen is sterile. You can do this by applying alcohol to the area. Then apply a two-percent iodine solution. Cover the clean area with a sterile four-by-four-inch gauze pad for two minutes.	☐	☐	☐
13. Now reapply the tourniquet. Ask the patient to make a fist. The maximum time the tourniquet should be in place is one minute.	☐	☐	☐
14. You're ready to penetrate the vein. It's easier to do if you hold the syringe or assembly in your dominant hand. Grasp the patient's arm with the other hand and use your thumb to draw the skin taut over the site.	☐	☐	☐
15. With the bevel up, line up the needle with the vein about one-fourth to one-half inch below the site where the vein is to be entered. Insert the needle into the vein at a 15- to 30-degree angle. Remove your nondominant hand and slowly pull back the plunger of the syringe. Or place fingers on the flange of the adapter	☐	☐	☐

	Self	Partner	Instructor
and with the thumb, push the tube onto the needle inside the adapter. When blood begins to flow into the tube or syringe, you can release the tourniquet and allow the patient to release the fist. Allow the syringe or tube to fill to capacity. When blood flow stops, remove the tube from the adapter by gripping the tube with your nondominant hand and placing your thumb against the flange during removal. Twist and gently pull out the tube. Hold the needle steady in the vein, without pulling up or pressing down, insert any other necessary tubes into the adapter, and fill each to capacity.			
16. Remove the tube from the adapter *before* removing the needle from the arm. This is important because you don't want any blood to drip from the tip of the needle onto the patient. Place a sterile gauze pad over the puncture site as you are withdrawing the needle.	☐	☐	☐
17. Apply pressure or have the patient apply direct pressure for five minutes. Don't let the patient bend the arm at the elbow.	☐	☐	☐
18. Transfer the blood from the syringe into the tubes using the proper order of draw. Always place the tubes in a tube rack to do the transfer. If the tubes contain an anticoagulant, you should mix immediately by gently inverting the tube eight to ten times. Do not shake the tube. Label the tubes with the proper information.	☐	☐	☐
19. Check the puncture site to be sure it isn't bleeding. Apply a dressing (a clean two-by-two inch gauze pad that you've folded in quarters). Secure it with an adhesive bandage or three-inch strip of tape.	☐	☐	☐
20. Thank your patient when you've finished. Tell your patient to leave the bandage in place for at least 30 minutes.	☐	☐	☐

Continued on back

	Self	Partner	Instructor
21. To finish your task, take care of or dispose of equipment and supplies. Clean your work area. Then you can remove your gloves and wash your hands.	☐	☐	☐
22. Test, transfer, or store the blood according to your office's policy.	☐	☐	☐
23. Record the procedure.	☐	☐	☐

Calculation

Total Possible Points: _____

Total Points Earned: _____ Multiplied by 100 = _____ Divided by Total Possible Points = _____ %

Pass   Fail   Comments:

☐   ☐

Student's signature _____ Date _____

Partner's signature _____ Date _____

Instructor's signature _____ Date _____

Hands On **Procedure 2-2:** Obtaining a Blood Specimen by Skin Puncture

Task: With a partner as the patient, obtain a blood specimen by skin puncture.

Conditions: The student will perform this task under the conditions described in the Procedure Steps, below.

Equipment/Supplies: sterile disposable lancet or automated skin puncture device; 70-percent alcohol or other antiseptic; sterile gauze pads; microcollection tubes or containers; heel-warming device (if necessary); biohazard barriers such as gloves, impervious gown, and face shield.

Standards: The student will perform this skill with _____ % accuracy in a total of _____ minutes. *(Your instructor will tell you what the percentage and time limits will be before you begin.)*

Key: 4 = Satisfactory   0 = Unsatisfactory   NA = this step is not counted

Procedure Steps	Self	Partner	Instructor
1. Check the requisition slip to see what tests have been ordered. Also note the specimen requirements.	☐	☐	☐
2. Assemble your equipment.	☐	☐	☐
3. Wash your hands.	☐	☐	☐
4. Greet and identify the patient. Explain the procedure and answer any questions.	☐	☐	☐
5. Put on gloves. Follow standard precautions.	☐	☐	☐
6. Select the puncture site. It will be one of the following: (A) just off center of the tip of the middle or ring finger of the nondominant hand (B) the lateral curved surface of the heel (C) the heel of an infant	☐	☐	☐
7. Make sure the site you've chosen is warm. Gently massage the finger from the base to the tip to increase blood flow.	☐	☐	☐

Continued on back

	Self	Partner	Instructor
8. You'll use both hands for this procedure. Grasp the finger or heel firmly with your nondominant hand. Now cleanse the area with alcohol and wipe dry.	☐	☐	☐
9. While you hold the finger or heel firmly, make a swift, firm puncture using your dominant hand. • After puncture, dispose of the used puncture device in a sharps container. • Wipe away the first drop of blood. It may be contaminated with tissue fluid or residue from your alcohol wipe. • Apply pressure toward the site.	☐	☐	☐
10. Collect the specimen. You can encourage blood flow by holding the puncture site downward and applying gentle pressure near the site.	☐	☐	☐
11. Once you've collected the blood you need, apply clean gauze to the site with pressure or have the patient apply pressure. Don't release your patient until the bleeding has stopped. Label the containers with the proper information.	☐	☐	☐
12. Thank your patient when you've finished. Tell your patient to leave the bandage in place for at least 30 minutes.	☐	☐	☐
13. To finish your task, take care of or dispose of equipment and supplies. Clean your work area. Then you can remove your gloves and wash your hands.	☐	☐	☐
14. Test, transfer, or store the specimen according to your office's policy, and record the procedure.	☐	☐	☐

Calculation

Total Possible Points: _____

Total Points Earned: _____ Multiplied by 100 = _____ Divided by Total Possible Points = _____ %

Pass   Fail   Comments:

☐   ☐

Student's signature _____ Date _____

Partner's signature _____ Date _____

Instructor's signature _____ Date _____

Chapter 3

HEMATOLOGY

Chapter Competencies

Review the information in your textbook that supports the following course objectives.

Before you begin studying, make sure you know the format of the test, for example, multiple choice, short answer, or essay questions. This will help you create a study plan.

Learning Objectives

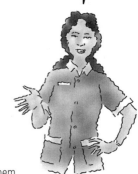

- Explain the functions of the three types of blood cells
- Identify the leukocytes normally seen in the blood and explain their functions
- Describe the role of the hematology lab
- List the different tests in a complete blood count
- Specify the normal ranges for each test in a complete blood count
- Use a Unopette system to prepare a whole blood dilution
- Make a peripheral blood smear
- Stain a peripheral blood smear
- Perform a white blood cell differential
- Describe the structure of red blood cells and explain the tests that are performed on them
- Perform a manual microhematocrit determination
- Determine a Westergren erythrocyte sedimentation rate
- Explain the functions of platelets
- Explain the process of how blood clots form in the body and describe the tests that measure the ability to form clots

Learning Self-Assessment Exercises

KEY TERMS

Use the clues to unscramble the following terms.

| T O | G Y | L O | M A | H E |

1. the study of blood and blood diseases

| O C | Y T | E S | U K | L E |

2. white blood cells

| E R | E S | Y T | Y T | O C | H R |

3. red blood cells

| O C | T H | M B | Y T | E S | R O |

4. platelets

| I A | E N | A M |

5. a condition resulting from a low number of red blood cells in the blood

| S T | A S | M O | H E | I S |

6. the body's ability to keep blood in a fluid state in the vessels

| O I | Y T | E T | H R | I N | O P | E R |

7. a hormone released from the kidneys that aids in the production of red blood cells

| I N | T H | O P | R O | M B | S T | L A |

8. a substance found in blood and tissues that aids the clotting process

| A | X I | P O | H Y |

9. a condition in which not enough oxygen reaches the body's tissues

| R | H E | T E | M O | T O | C Y | M E |

10. the manual counting chamber used to count each type of blood cell

| M A | I S | T O | H E | E S | P O |

11. production of blood cells

| M O | H E | G L | I N | O B |

12. the protein in red blood cells that transports oxygen from the lungs to the tissues

| M O | N O | T E | C Y |

13. a large white blood cell that surrounds and absorbs microorganisms and other foreign bodies in the blood and tissues

M	P	L Y	H O	C Y	T E

_____

14. a type of white blood cell (WBC) that plays a part in the body's development of immunity

N E	U T	I L	R O	P H

_____

15. a type of white blood cell that is highly destructive of microorganisms

PROCEDURE PRACTICE

Below is a sequence chart for staining a peripheral blood smear. Fill in the missing steps with the choices from the answer bank on the next page.

> Many of the terms you need to learn sound similar. Creating flash cards to help you memorize vocabulary might help you memorize unfamiliar terms.

1. _____

↓

2. _____

_____

↓

3. Greet and identify the patient. Explain the procedure. Ask for and answer any questions.

↓

4. Put on gloves, an impervious gown, and a face shield.

↓

5. _____

_____

_____

↓

6. Label the slide with the patient's name or identification number on the frosted area using a pencil.

↓

7. _____

_____

↓

8. Use the thumb and forefinger on your dominant hand to hold the second (spreader) slide against the surface of the first slide at a 30-degree angle.

- The angle of the spreader slide may have to be greater for large or thin drops of blood.
- The angle of the spreader slide may have to be less than 20 degrees for small or thick drops.

Move the spreader slide back until it is touching the drop of blood. Allow the blood to spread under the edge for a fraction of a second. Then push the spreader slide at a medium speed toward the other end of the slide. Make sure the two slides are in contact the entire time.

↓

9. _____

↓

10. _____

ANSWER BANK

➤ Hold the slide flat between the thumb and first finger on your nondominant hand. Place a drop of blood 1 cm from the frosting at one end of the slide. The slide also can be held on a flat surface and the smear made on the surface. Try both ways and see which is more comfortable and gets the best results.

➤ Wash your hands.

➤ Properly take care of or dispose of equipment and supplies. Clean your work area. Then, remove your gloves, gown, and face shield, and wash your hands.

➤ Perform a venipuncture to get an EDTA (lavender-top tube) blood specimen from your patient.

➤ Allow the slide to air dry.

➤ Get your equipment ready.

LABELING

Identify the different types of blood cells shown in the diagram.

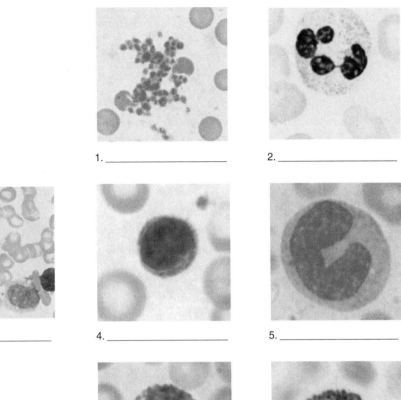

1. _____

2. _____

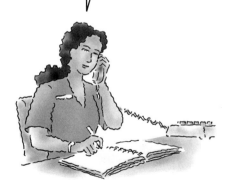

3. _____

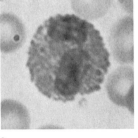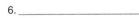

4. _____

5. _____

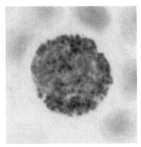

6. _____

7. _____

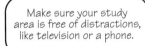

Make sure your study
area is free of distractions,
like television or a phone.

PRACTICE QUIZ

1. The body's main line of defense against bacteria and viruses are:
   a. platelets.
   b. hemoglobin.
   c. leukocytes.
   d. erythrocytes.

2. Which of the following will not lead to leukocytosis?
   a. infection
   b. poor nutrition
   c. injury to tissue
   d. inflammatory condition

3. Blood cells can form in all of the following body parts except the:
   a. heart.
   b. liver.
   c. skull.
   d. long bones.

4. Which of the following could happen to a person with a lower-than-normal platelet count?
   a. increased clotting
   b. increased bleeding
   c. lack of oxygen to cells
   d. severe bacterial infection

5. What is the benefit of adding a stain to white blood cells on a slide?
   a. The stain removes the hemoglobin from the cells.
   b. The stain marks the cells that are infected with a virus.
   c. The stain blocks the cells from carrying out their job.
   d. The stain lets you see the cells since they are colorless.

6. A condition that results from a reduced number of red blood cells in the blood is called:
   a. anemia.
   b. hematopoiesis.
   c. leukemia.
   d. microcytosis.

7. What percentage of the normal white blood cells do segmented neutrophils make up?
   a. 0–5%
   b. 3–8%
   c. 20–40%
   d. 50–70%

8. What is the main function of red blood cells?
   a. form blood clots
   b. fight off infections
   c. bring nutrients to the cells
   d. carry gases between the lungs and the body tissues

9. Which of the following statements about blood cells is TRUE?
   a. A mature red blood cell has no nucleus.
   b. Neutrophils help to transport oxygen to cells.
   c. A white blood cell is also called an erythrocyte.
   d. The lymphocyte is the most common type of white blood cell.

10. Which of the following can be discovered through hematology testing?
    a. how energy is used to break down food
    b. the amount of blood cells produced in the bone marrow
    c. how many blood cells are pumped by the heart every second
    d. problems related to abnormal growth of bone marrow

CRITICAL THINKING PRACTICE

Blood Samples and Tests

Review these scenarios below and answer the questions that follow.

1. Maria arrived late to work and is behind on running blood tests. She enters the lab, washes her hands, and grabs a blood collection tube with a standard rubber stopper. When she opens the tube, aerosols are released into the air. She may have just exposed herself to harmful pathogens. What are two things Maria could have done to protect herself?

   A. _____

   _____

   B. _____

   _____

2. The new medical assistant is trying to prepare a slide of white cells for a white blood cell count and differential. He asks you for help because after three attempts he still cannot see the white blood cells. What should you tell him?

   _____

   _____

   _____

   _____

Coumadin Therapy

A patient in your office has been put on the drug Coumadin because he had a heart attack. The patient will need to go for routine prothrombin time blood tests as a result of being on this medication. The physician has asked you to explain the medication to the patient.
   Decide if each statement is true or false. If it is false, what can you do to correct it?

1. Coumadin is used for the immediate prevention of new clot formation.

   True   False

   _____

   _____

2. The prothrombin time test will measure clotting in the blood.

   True   False

   _____

   _____

3. If your Coumadin dosage is too low, you may experience excessive bleeding.

   True   False

   _____

   _____

Certification Prep

1. What blood cells are formed in the bone marrow and are important in blood clotting?
   a. leukocytes
   b. thrombocytes
   c. monocytes
   d. neutrophils

2. What is the measurement of packed red blood cells (RBCs) in relation to the total blood volume called?
   a. hemoglobin
   b. complete blood count (CBC)
   c. hematocrit
   d. erythrocyte sedimentation rate (ESR)

3. When clotting has not been allowed and the tube is centrifuged, what is the clear liquid that appears called?
   a. plasma
   b. erythrocytes
   c. serum
   d. buffy coat

4. What is one of the main functions of white blood cells (WBCs)?
   a. carry oxygen to the brain
   b. transport glucose across the cell membrane
   c. defend against viruses and bacteria
   d. monitor the clotting factor

5. What are monocytes?
   a. single-cell proteins, a by-product of glycogen synthesis
   b. the largest leukocytes in the circulating blood
   c. bacteria that cause mononucleosis
   d. assist in platelet formation

6. What does a CBC include?
   a. RBC, WBC, bleeding time, and sedimentation rate
   b. RBC, WBC, hemoglobin, and sedimentation rate
   c. RBC, WBC, hematocrit, and hemoglobin
   d. WBC, bleeding time, RBC, and hemoglobin

7. What is a test called that breaks down the percentage of each type of WBC?
   a. WBC
   b. ESR
   c. PTT/INR
   d. differential

8. The term leukopenia means:
   a. decreased white cells.
   b. enlarged white cells.
   c. increased thrombocytes.
   d. increased white cells.

9. Drugs that prevent the formation of clots are classified as:
   a. antiemetics.
   b. antipyretics.
   c. antineoplastics.
   d. anticoagulants.

Name _____ Date _____ Time _____

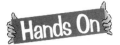 **Procedure 3-1:** Preparing a Whole Blood Dilution
Using the Unopette System

Task: Prepare a whole blood dilution using the Unopette system.

Conditions: The student will perform this task under the conditions described in the Procedure Steps, below.

Equipment/Supplies: Unopette system; gauze

Standards: The student will perform this skill with ____ % accuracy in a total of ____ minutes. *(Your instructor will tell you what the percentage and time limits will be before you begin.)*

Key: 4 = Satisfactory   0 = Unsatisfactory   NA = this step is not counted

Procedure Steps	Self	Partner	Instructor
1. Wash your hands.	☐	☐	☐
2. Get your equipment ready. Put on gloves, gown, and face shield.	☐	☐	☐
3. Pierce the diaphragm in the neck of the plastic reservoir. • Push the tip of the shield on the capillary pipette through the diaphragm. • When you insert the shield, use a twisting motion. • Then, remove the outer protective shield from the pipette.	☐	☐	☐
4. Fill the pipette with free-flowing whole blood. • You may get the blood by performing a skin puncture or from a well-mixed lavender top tube specimen. • If filling from a tube, place the tip of the Unopette just below the surface of the blood. Allow capillary action to fill the tube completely.	☐	☐	☐
5. Wipe the pipette with gauze or lab tissue to remove excess blood, but be careful not to wipe across the pipette's tip. This is because the gauze could absorb some of the blood sample and cause false test results.	☐	☐	☐

Continued on back

	Self	Partner	Instructor
6. Gently squeeze the reservoir to help expel some of the air. Make sure you don't push out any of the diluting fluids. Getting some of the air out of the reservoir will help create a vacuum that will help when filling the unit.	☐	☐	☐
7. Cover the opposite end of the pipette from where the blood came in with your finger. Keeping pressure on the sides of the reservoir, insert the pipette through the hole previously made in the diaphragm until the lower collar on the pipette makes a seal with the neck on the reservoir.	☐	☐	☐
8. Once you have achieved a seal, remove your finger from the end of the pipette and simultaneously release the pressure exerted on the sides of the reservoir.	☐	☐	☐
9. Gently squeeze and release the reservoir several times to force the diluting fluids just slightly into but not out of the pipette's overflow chamber.	☐	☐	☐
10. Put your index finger over the opening of the pipette's overflow chamber and gently turn it upside down or swirl the container several times to mix. Remove the pipette, invert it, and insert it back into the neck of the reservoir with the pipette sticking out. Next, cover the pipette with the plastic protective cover removed earlier. You can place the whole reservoir-pipette assembly on a blood rocker, if one is available.	☐	☐	☐
11. Carefully label the specimen with all the required information.	☐	☐	☐

Calculation

Total Possible Points: _____

Total Points Earned: _____ Multiplied by 100 = _____ Divided by Total Possible Points = _____ %

Pass   Fail   Comments:

☐   ☐

Student's signature _____ Date _____

Partner's signature _____ Date _____

Instructor's signature _____ Date _____

Hands On — **Procedure 3-2:** Making a Peripheral Blood Smear

Task: With a partner as the patient, perform a venipuncture and then make a peripheral blood smear.

Conditions: The student will perform this task under the conditions described in the Procedure Steps, below.

Equipment/Supplies: clean glass slides with frosted ends; a pencil; a well-mixed whole blood specimen; a transfer pipette

Standards: The student will perform this skill with _____ % accuracy in a total of _____ minutes. *(Your instructor will tell you what the percentage and time limits will be before you begin.)*

Key: 4 = Satisfactory   0 = Unsatisfactory   NA = this step is not counted

Procedure Steps	Self	Partner	Instructor
1. Wash your hands.	☐	☐	☐
2. Get your equipment ready.	☐	☐	☐
3. Greet and identify the patient. Explain the procedure. Ask for and answer any questions.	☐	☐	☐
4. Put on gloves, an impervious gown, and a face shield.	☐	☐	☐
5. Perform a venipuncture as described in Chapter 2 to get an EDTA (lavender-top tube) blood specimen from your patient.	☐	☐	☐
6. Label the slide with the patient's name or identification number on the frosted area using a pencil.	☐	☐	☐
7. Hold the slide flat between the thumb and first finger on your nondominant hand. Place a drop of blood 1 cm from the frosting at one end of the slide. The slide also can be held on a flat surface and the smear made on the surface. Try both ways and see which is more comfortable and gets the best results.	☐	☐	☐

Continued on back

	Self	Partner	Instructor
8. Use your thumb and forefinger on your dominant hand to hold the second (spreader) slide against the surface of the first slide at a 30-degree angle. • The angle of the spreader slide may have to be greater for large or thin drops of blood. • The angle of the spreader slide may have to be less than 30 degrees for small or thick drops. Move the spreader slide back until it is touching the drop of blood. Allow the blood to spread under the edge for a fraction of a second. Then push the spreader slide at a medium speed toward the other end of the slide. Make sure the two slides are in contact the entire time.	☐	☐	☐
9. Allow the slide to air dry.	☐	☐	☐
10. Properly take care of or dispose of equipment and supplies. Clean your work area. Then, remove your gloves, gown, and face shield, and wash your hands.	☐	☐	☐

Calculation

Total Possible Points: _____

Total Points Earned: _____ Multiplied by 100 = _____ Divided by Total Possible Points = _____ %

Pass   Fail   Comments:

☐   ☐

Student's signature _____ Date _____

Partner's signature _____ Date _____

Instructor's signature _____ Date _____

Name _____ Date _____ Time _____

🪶 Hands On 🪶 Procedure 3-3: Staining a Peripheral Blood Smear

Task: Stain a peripheral blood smear using Giemsa stain and water or a Wright's buffer.

Conditions: The student will perform this task under the conditions described in the Procedure Steps, below.

Equipment/Supplies: a staining rack; Wright's stain; Giemsa stain; a prepared slide; tweezers

Standards: The student will perform this skill with _____ % accuracy in a total of _____ minutes. *(Your instructor will tell you what the percentage and time limits will be before you begin.)*

Key: 4 = Satisfactory   0 = Unsatisfactory   NA = this step is not counted

Procedure Steps	Self	Partner	Instructor
1. Wash your hands.	☐	☐	☐
2. Get your equipment ready.	☐	☐	☐
3. Put on gloves, an impervious gown, and a face shield.	☐	☐	☐
4. Get the dried blood smear. Keep in mind that a smear made from blood that's more than four hours old may have deteriorated cells.	☐	☐	☐
5. Place the slide on a stain rack, blood side up. Then, flood the slide with Wright's stain. Leave the stain on the slide for three to five minutes or for the time specified by the manufacturer. The alcohol in Wright's stain helps fix the blood to the slide.	☐	☐	☐
6. Use your tweezers to tilt the slide so that the stain drains off. Then, apply equal amounts of Giemsa stain and water or a Wright's buffer. A green sheen will appear on the slide's surface. Let the solution remain on the slide for five minutes or the time specified by the manufacturer. This helps improve the quality of the stain.	☐	☐	☐

Continued on back

	Self	Partner	Instructor
7. Again, hold the slide with your tweezers. Gently rinse the slide with water to remove any excess stain. Wipe off the back of the slide with gauze. Stand the slide upright and allow it to dry.	☐	☐	☐
8. Properly take care of or dispose of equipment and supplies. Clean your work area. Then, remove your gloves, gown, and face shield, and wash your hands.	☐	☐	☐

Calculation

Total Possible Points: _____

Total Points Earned: _____ Multiplied by 100 = _____ Divided by Total Possible Points = _____ %

Pass   Fail   Comments:

☐   ☐

Student's signature _____ Date _____

Partner's signature _____ Date _____

Instructor's signature _____ Date _____

Name _____ Date _____ Time _____

Hands On Procedure 3-4: Performing a White Blood Cell Differential

Task: Perform a white blood cell differential.

Conditions: The student will perform this task under the conditions described in the Procedure Steps, below.

Equipment/Supplies: a stained peripheral blood smear; a microscope; immersion oil; paper; a recording tabulator (differential calculator)

Standards: The student will perform this skill with _____ % accuracy in a total of _____ minutes. *(Your instructor will tell you what the percentage and time limits will be before you begin.)*

Key: 4 = Satisfactory   0 = Unsatisfactory   NA = this step is not counted

Procedure Steps	Self	Partner	Instructor
1. Wash your hands.	☐	☐	☐
2. Get your equipment ready. Put on gloves.	☐	☐	☐
3. Put the stained slide on the microscope. Focus on the feathered edge of the smear and scan with the low-power objective to make sure the cells are evenly distributed and properly stained.	☐	☐	☐
4. Carefully turn the nosepiece to the high-power objective and bring the slide into focus using the fine adjustment.	☐	☐	☐
5. Carefully turn the nosepiece so the point of focus on the slide is between the high-power objective and the oil objective.	☐	☐	☐
6. Place a drop of oil on the slide and move the oil immersion lens into place using the fine adjustment. Focus and begin to identify any leukocytes. (The oil helps to provide a path for the light between the specimen on the slide and the oil immersion objective.)	☐	☐	☐

Continued on back

	Self	Partner	Instructor
7. Record on a tally sheet or differential counter the types of white cells you find. This way, you'll be able to calculate accurate percentages.	☐	☐	☐
8. Move the stage so the next field is in view. Identify any white cells in this field and then continue to the next field. The goal is to view as many fields as necessary to count 100 white cells. Move the stage systematically so you know where you counted and where you still need to count, to find new cells, and to avoid counting the same cell twice.	☐	☐	☐
9. Record the number of each type of leukocyte (WBC) as a percentage. Remember that because you counted 100 cells, each cell represents one percentage point.	☐	☐	☐
10. Properly take care of or dispose of equipment and supplies. Clean your work area. Then, remove your gloves and wash your hands.	☐	☐	☐

Calculation

Total Possible Points: _____

Total Points Earned: _____ Multiplied by 100 = _____ Divided by Total Possible Points = _____ %

Pass   Fail   Comments:

☐   ☐

Student's signature _____ Date _____

Partner's signature _____ Date _____

Instructor's signature _____ Date _____

Name _____ Date _____ Time _____

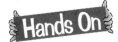 **Procedure 3-5:** Performing a Manual Microhematocrit Determination

Task: Perform a manual microhematocrit determination from a capillary puncture and from an EDTA tube of whole blood.

Conditions: The student will perform this task under the conditions described in the Procedure Steps, below.

Equipment/Supplies: microcollection tubes; sealing clay; a microhematocrit centrifuge; a microhematocrit reading device

Standards: The student will perform this skill with _____ % accuracy in a total of _____ minutes. *(Your instructor will tell you what the percentage and time limits will be before you begin.)*

Key: 4 = Satisfactory   0 = Unsatisfactory   NA = this step is not counted

Procedure Steps	Self	Partner	Instructor
1. Wash your hands.	☐	☐	☐
2. Get your equipment ready.	☐	☐	☐
3. Put on gloves, a gown, and a face shield.	☐	☐	☐
4. Use one of the following methods to draw blood into the capillary tube. A. *Directly from a capillary puncture:* • Touch the tip of the capillary tube to the blood at the wound and allow to fill to three-quarters or the indicated mark. • For a finger stick, use heparinized capillary tubes. • Place your forefinger over the top of the capillary tube, wipe excess blood off its sides, and push its bottom into the sealing clay. (Make sure you push the end opposite to the end the blood was drawn in.) Use caution while sealing tubes as they can break and puncture gloves and skin if you use too much force. • Then, draw a second specimen in the same way. (The second tube is for a duplicate test as a part of quality control.)	☐	☐	☐

Continued on back

	Self	Partner	Instructor
B. *From a well-mixed EDTA tube of whole blood:* • Touch the tip of the capillary tube to the blood in the EDTA tube and allow the capillary tube to fill three-quarters. • Place your forefinger over the top of the capillary tube, wipe excess blood off its sides, and push its bottom into the sealing clay. (Make sure you push the end opposite to the end the blood was drawn in.) Use caution while sealing tubes as they can break and puncture gloves and skin if you use too much force. • Then, draw a second specimen in the same way. (The second tube is for a duplicate test as a part of quality control.)			
5. Place the tubes, with the clay-sealed end out, in the radial grooves of the microhematocrit centrifuge opposite each other. Put the lid on the grooved area and tighten by turning the knob clockwise. Close the lid. Spin for five minutes or as directed by the manufacturer.	☐	☐	☐
6. Remove the tubes from the centrifuge and read the results. Instructions on how to do this are printed on the device. Take the average and report it as a percentage. (The figure shows the determinations of microhematocrit values. Results should be within two percent of each other. Results that have greater than a two-percent variation are unreliable. A three-percent difference is the equivalent of a patient losing about a pint of blood.)	☐	☐	☐
7. Dispose of the microhematocrit tubes in a biohazard container. Properly take care of or dispose of other equipment and supplies. Clean your work area. Then, remove your gloves, gown, and face shield, and wash your hands.	☐	☐	☐

Calculation

Total Possible Points: _____

Total Points Earned: _____ Multiplied by 100 = _____ Divided by Total Possible Points = _____ %

Pass   Fail   Comments:

☐   ☐

Student's signature _____ Date _____

Partner's signature _____ Date _____

Instructor's signature _____ Date _____

Name _____ Date _____ Time _____

Hands On **Procedure 3-6:** Performing a Westergren Erythrocyte
Sedimentation Rate

Task: Perform a Westergren Erythrocyte Sedimentation Rate.

Conditions: The student will perform this task under the conditions described in the Procedure Steps, below.

Equipment/Supplies: a whole blood sample collected in EDTA (free of clots and less than four hours old); a Sediplast system vial prefilled with 0.2 mL of 3.8 percent sodium citrate; an autozero calibrated Sediplast pipette; a sedrate rack; a disposable transfer pipette

Standards: The student will perform this skill with _____ % accuracy in a total of _____ minutes. *(Your instructor will tell you what the percentage and time limits will be before you begin.)*

Key: 4 = Satisfactory   0 = Unsatisfactory   NA = this step is not counted

Procedure Steps	Self	Partner	Instructor
1. Wash your hands.	☐	☐	☐
2. Get your equipment ready.	☐	☐	☐
3. Put on gloves, gown, and face shield.	☐	☐	☐
4. Remove the stopper on the prefilled vial. Using a transfer pipette, fill the vial to the bottom of the indicated fill line with 0.8 mL of blood to make the required 4:1 dilution. (The test can also be run with no dilution.)	☐	☐	☐
5. Replace the pierceable stopper and gently invert several times. This way, there will be a good mixture of blood and diluent.	☐	☐	☐
6. Place the vial in its rack on a level surface. Carefully insert the pipette through the pierceable stopper using a rotating downward pressure until the pipette comes in contact with the bottom of the vial. The pipette will autozero the blood and any excess will flow into the reservoir compartment.	☐	☐	☐

Continued on back

	Self	Partner	Instructor
7. Make sure the pipette makes firm contact with the bottom of the vial. Otherwise, you may get inaccurate test results.	☐	☐	☐
8. Let the sample stand for exactly one hour and then read the numerical results of the erythrocyte sedimentation in millimeters. Make sure the test is set up on a surface that is free from vibration and away from anything that may cause a change in temperature (windows, refrigerators, motors, AC ducts). Most of these will cause an increase in sedimentation rate, but cold will cause a decrease.	☐	☐	☐
9. Properly take care of or dispose of equipment and supplies. Clean your work area. Then remove your gloves, gown, and face shield and wash your hands.	☐	☐	☐

Calculation

Total Possible Points: _____

Total Points Earned: _____ Multiplied by 100 = _____ Divided by Total Possible Points = _____ %

Pass   Fail   Comments:

☐   ☐

Student's signature _____ Date _____

Partner's signature _____ Date _____

Instructor's signature _____ Date _____

Chapter 4

IMMUNOLOGY AND IMMUNOHEMATOLOGY

Chapter Competencies

Review the information in your textbook that supports the following course objectives.

> Try organizing some of your notes into tables, charts, and other formats. Sometimes a concept might be easier to understand if you look at it from a different perspective.

Learning Objectives

- Describe the different types of immunity
- Identify the different types of antibodies
- List the reasons for immunological testing
- Describe the antigen-antibody reaction
- Explain the principles of agglutination testing and ELISA
- Summarize the proper storage and handling of immunology test kits
- Describe the ways that quality control is applied to immunology testing
- List and describe immunology tests most commonly performed in the medical office or physician office lab
- Perform an HCG pregnancy test
- Perform a Group A rapid strep test
- Identify the major blood types and explain why differences in blood type exist
- Describe how blood is typed and explain why this testing is important

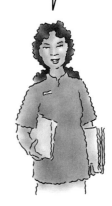

Learning Self-Assessment Exercises

KEY TERMS

Complete the crossword puzzle below with the appropriate key terms, using the clues on the next page.

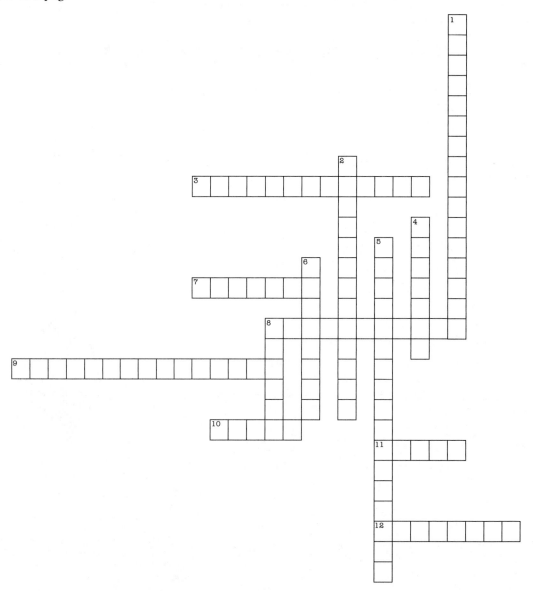

ACROSS

3. the clumping together of particles, red blood cells, or bacteria, usually in response to the presence of antibodies
7. protein markers on cells that cause formation of antibodies and that react specifically with those antibodies
8. design of antibody to recognize and bind with only one antigen
9. a solution that is tested the same way as a patient's sample and its expected result is already known
10. the concentration amount of an antibody in serum
11. a person who contributes blood
12. protein produced by the body to fight non-self substance

DOWN

1. testing performed by blood banks on red blood cells and serum to make sure the donor blood matches the person receiving it
2. test result that says a substance is present in a specimen when it actually is not
4. having excess fat in the blood
5. a disease caused by antibodies that attack its own cells or tissues
6. control tools built into a serology test kit to ensure that test procedures are followed correctly and that reagents are working properly
8. a solution of sodium chloride and sterile water commonly used in IV infusions

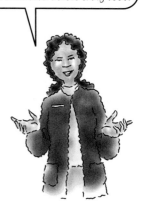

If you don't feel comfortable asking your questions in the class, ask the teacher after class or during office hours. Just make sure you get your questions answered before a big test!

PROCEDURE PRACTICE

Performing an HCG Pregnancy Test

Follow the appropriate procedure for performing an HCG pregnancy test. For each step that appears below, write C if the step is correct or I if it is incorrect. If a step is incorrect, briefly describe the correct process.

_____ **1.** Wash your hands.

_____

_____ **2.** Assemble the test kit's equipment. The kit should be warmed to 92°F.

_____

_____ **3.** Check that the names on the specimen container and lab form are the same.

_____

_____ 4. Use two test packs for the patient and two for each control.

_____

_____ 5. Label the three test packs as follows: the patient's name, "test 1," and "test 2."

_____

_____ 6. In the patient's chart and the control log, record the type of specimen you're obtaining (urine or plasma/serum).

_____

_____ 7. Carefully aspirate the positive control and place four drops in the sample well of the pack labeled "positive control."

_____

_____ 8. Use a transfer pipette to aspirate the specimen. Place four drops in the sample well of the test pack labeled with the patient's name.

_____

_____ 9. Follow the exact same step for the negative control.

_____

_____ 10. Consult the test manufacturer's insert in the kit to interpret test results. The insert will tell you what to look for in reading a positive or negative result.

_____

_____ 11. Report the results when the end-of-assay window is read and after you have checked the controls for accuracy. This will happen at about one minute for serum and about eight minutes for urine.

_____

_____ 12. Record the controls and patient's information on the worksheet or log form and in the patient's records.

_____

_____ 13. Clean up the work area and dispose of all waste properly.

_____

Labeling Blood Types

Fill in the missing information in the table about blood group donors and recipients. Then answer the questions that follow.

Blood Group Donors and Recipients

Blood Group	Antigens	Antibodies	Can Receive Blood from	Can Give Blood to
A	A	Anti-B	_____	A, AB
B	B	_____	_____	B, AB
AB	_____	None	_____	_____
O	_____	_____	O	_____

1. Why is a person with type O blood considered a "universal donor"?

   _____

   _____

2. Why is it important to know a person's blood type?

   _____

   _____

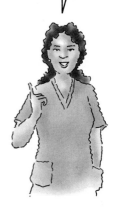

If you're easily distracted while studying in a busy place, try wearing ear plugs to block out the noise.

PRACTICE QUIZ

1. Immunology tests are carried out on which component of the blood?
   a. serum
   b. platelets
   c. buffy coat
   d. red blood cells

2. Agglutination results in which the solution appears smooth and milky are:
   a. negative.
   b. positive.
   c. false-negative.
   d. false-positive.

3. Which of the following is an example of active induced immunity?
   a. getting a vaccine
   b. coming down with a virus
   c. getting antibodies from the mother while nursing
   d. receiving already made antibodies as part of therapy

4. All of the following statements about antibodies are TRUE except:
   a. antibodies are specific.
   b. antibodies are proteins.
   c. antibodies have a very weak attraction to their antigens.
   d. antibodies are named after the specific antigen they are attracted to and by adding the prefix anti-.

5. What determines a person's blood type?
   a. the type of antibodies produced
   b. the amount of platelets in the blood
   c. the type of antigens on the red blood cells
   d. the type of antigens on the white blood cells

6. Which of the following statements about antigens is TRUE?
   a. Foreign antigens cause antibodies to be produced.
   b. They enter the body from an outside source.
   c. Antigens that determine blood type are found in white blood cells.
   d. Bacteria and viruses only have antigens once inside a human body.

7. The most common blood group in the United States is:
   a. Type A.
   b. Type B.
   c. Type AB.
   d. Type O.

8. Rob's blood has an A antigen, a B antigen, and a D antigen. What type of blood does he have?
   a. AB negative
   b. AB positive
   c. O negative
   d. O positive

9. "The first antibody to respond to antigens" and "it doesn't cross the placental barrier" are characteristics that describe:
   a. immunoglobin A.
   b. immunoglobin E.
   c. immunoglobin G.
   d. immunoglobin M.

10. Which of the following would help to avoid false-positive or false-negative results?
    a. only use lipemic blood samples
    b. follow directions carefully when conducting a test
    c. wait double the recommended time to look for agglutination
    d. use blood samples in which the red blood cell membranes have ruptured

CRITICAL THINKING

Using Reagents

Read the following guidelines about reagent use below. Mark each statement *True* or *False* and explain how each false statement could be corrected.

1. All reagents should be stored in the refrigerator for best quality.

    True   False

    _____

    _____

2. Never use a reagent after the expiration date.

    True   False

    _____

    _____

3. When you open a new test kit, write the date because some kits have a new expiration date that starts from the day they are opened.

    True   False

    _____

    _____

4. If you accidentally add another solution to the reagent, the reagent should be discarded because it might not work properly.

    True   False

    _____

    _____

5. Each reagent kit is marked with a lot number. It is okay to use reagents with different lot numbers.

    True   False

    _____

    _____

6. Always read the kit's package insert for details about handling its reagents and supplies.

    True   False

    _____

    _____

7. Do not use reagents that were shipped against the normal guidelines.

   True   False

   _____

   _____

Active and Passive Immunity

There are different ways a person can develop immunity. Identify each of the following statements as active (A) or passive (P) immunity.

_____ 1. A woman comes down with the flu and develops antibodies to it.

_____ 2. A nursing infant receives antibodies from its mother.

_____ 3. A toddler gets a vaccine for the measles.

_____ 4. A ten-year-old gets chickenpox. Years later he is exposed to chickenpox but does not develop it.

_____ 5. Antibodies cross the placenta from mother to fetus.

Certification Prep

1. What is a particular challenge of being an organ transplant recipient?
   a. The recipient's immune response is blocked.
   b. When antigens are foreign, or other than "self," the body attempts to destroy them.
   c. The individual's immune response builds antibodies against "self" antigens.
   d. Immune globulin is neutralized.

2. What is immunity acquired from another source called, such as that transferred across the placenta from mother to fetus?
   a. passive acquired natural immunity
   b. inactive acquired artificial immunity
   c. active acquired artificial immunity
   d. active acquired natural immunity

3. What are proteins called that are produced by plasma cells in response to foreign antigens and that provide immediate antibody protection that lasts for weeks?
   a. immune globulins
   b. toxoids
   c. interferon
   d. B lymphocytes

4. What are some of the major problems facing the American Red Cross and other blood banks?
   a. lack of facilities where people may come to donate blood
   b. shortage of qualified, detail-oriented staff members
   c. obtaining sufficient amounts of safe blood and blood products to meet patients' needs
   d. too many regulatory guidelines that must be met in order to assure quality control

5. Which statement is NOT an indicator of why a false-positive or false-negative may occur?
   a. if testing personnel wait too long to read agglutination
   b. because testing personnel control the biologic conditions
   c. because of technical difficulty with samples
   d. because of technical difficulty performing the test

6. Why might a pregnancy test be ordered, even when the woman believes she is not pregnant?
   a. negative result helps rule out hormone imbalance
   b. it is part of a woman's routine annual physical exam
   c. to rule out pregnancy before performing medical procedures that might harm a fetus
   d. helps differentiate between pregnancy and early menopause

7. What is true about the "shelf life" of plasma?
   a. Plasma has a very short shelf life of 30 days.
   b. Plasma can be refrigerated for one year.
   c. Plasma can be frozen for one year.
   d. Plasma remains usable as long as it has no visible color change.

8. What is the best reason kits should be tested periodically for continued stability of all reagents?
   a. It's part of a good quality control policy.
   b. It shows your concern for accuracy.
   c. Reagents do not always function properly even before the expiration date.
   d. The products may be inferior and you need to know whether to buy more of the same.

9. How are platelet concentrates used?
   a. as a diluent for certain powdered intravenous medications
   b. to replace blood products when the patient is too hypertensive to take on whole blood
   c. to replace blood volume if blood pressure is too low
   d. to treat bleeding because of low-platelet count or dysfunctional platelets

10. What is immunohematology?
    a. tests that are based on the attraction between platelets and pathogens
    b. testing done in blood banks on red blood cells and serum
    c. means the donor's blood is compatible with a recipient's blood
    d. tests to see if an individual will benefit from transfusions

Name _____ Date _____ Time _____

Hands On   Procedure 4-1: Performing an HCG Pregnancy Test

Task: Perform an HCG pregnancy test.

Conditions: The student will perform this task under the conditions described in the Procedure Steps, below.

Equipment/Supplies: test kit; patient's chart; control log; transfer pipette

Standards: The student will perform this skill with _____ % accuracy in a total of _____ minutes. *(Your instructor will tell you what the percentage and time limits will be before you begin.)*

Key: 4 = Satisfactory   0 = Unsatisfactory   NA = this step is not counted

Procedure Steps	Self	Partner	Instructor
1. Wash your hands.	☐	☐	☐
2. Assemble the test kit's equipment. The kit should be at room temperature.	☐	☐	☐
3. Check that the names on the specimen container and lab form are the same.	☐	☐	☐
4. Use one test pack for the patient and one for each control.	☐	☐	☐
5. Label the three test packs as follows: the patient's name, "positive control," and "negative control."	☐	☐	☐
6. In the patient's chart and the control log, record the type of specimen you're obtaining (urine or plasma/serum).	☐	☐	☐
7. Use a transfer pipette to aspirate the specimen. Place four drops in the sample well of the test pack labeled with the patient's name.	☐	☐	☐
8. Carefully aspirate the positive control and place four drops in the sample well of the pack labeled "positive control."	☐	☐	☐

Continued on back

	Self	Partner	Instructor
9. Follow the exact same step for the negative control.	☐	☐	☐
10. Consult the test manufacturer's insert in the kit to interpret test results. The insert will tell you what to look for in reading a positive or negative control.	☐	☐	☐
11. Report the results when the end-of-assay window is read and after you have checked the controls for accuracy. This will happen at about seven minutes for serum and about four minutes for urine. The end-of-assay window should either change or appear wet. If it does not and/or the controls do not work, the rest must be redone.	☐	☐	☐
12. Record the controls and patient's information on the worksheet or log form and in the patient's records.	☐	☐	☐
13. Clean up the work area and dispose of all waste properly.	☐	☐	☐

Calculation

Total Possible Points: _____

Total Points Earned: _____ Multiplied by 100 = _____ Divided by Total Possible Points = _____ %

Pass   Fail   Comments:

☐   ☐

Student's signature _____ Date _____

Partner's signature _____ Date _____

Instructor's signature _____ Date _____

Name _____ Date _____ Time _____

Task: Perform a Group A rapid strep test.

Conditions: The student will perform this task under the conditions described in the Procedure Steps, below.

Equipment/Supplies: test kit; specimem container; timer

Standards: The student will perform this skill with _____ % accuracy in a total of _____ minutes. *(Your instructor will tell you what the percentage and time limits will be before you begin.)*

Key: 4 = Satisfactory   0 = Unsatisfactory   NA = this step is not counted

Procedure Steps	Self	Partner	Instructor
1. Wash your hands.	☐	☐	☐
2. Double check that the names on the specimen container and the lab form are the same.	☐	☐	☐
3. Label one extraction tube with the patient's name, one with "positive control," and one with "negative control."	☐	☐	☐
4. Follow the kit directions. Carefully add the correct reagents and drops to each of the extraction tubes.	☐	☐	☐
5. Insert the patient's culture swab (which is one of the two swabs) into the labeled extraction tube. If only one swab was taken, first swab a beta strep agar plate. Then, use the same swab for the actual test.	☐	☐	☐
6. Add the right controls to each of the two control tubes and place a sterile swab into each control tube.	☐	☐	☐
7. Use the swab to mix each tube's contents by twirling each swab five to six times.	☐	☐	☐

Continued on back

	Self	Partner	Instructor
8. Set a timer for the amount of time specified by the manufacturer of the test.	☐	☐	☐
9. Draw the swab up from the bottom on each tube and out of any liquid. Press out all fluid on the swab head by rolling the swab against the inside of the tube before it is withdrawn.	☐	☐	☐
10. Add three drops from the well-mixed extraction tube to the sample window of the strep A test unit labeled with the patient's name. Do the same for each control.	☐	☐	☐
11. Set the timer for the correct amount of time.	☐	☐	☐
12. A positive result will show up as a line in the result window within five minutes.	☐	☐	☐
13. A negative result is indicated if no line appears within five minutes. However, you must wait exactly five minutes to read a negative result, to avoid getting a false-negative.	☐	☐	☐
14. Verify the control results before recording any test results. Log the controls and the patient's information into your log or worksheet.	☐	☐	☐
15. You may have to culture all negative rapid strep tests on a blood agar if your lab requires it. (A bacteria disk may be added to the first quadrant when you set up the blood agar.)	☐	☐	☐
16. Clean up the work area and dispose of all waste in the right place.	☐	☐	☐
17. Don't forget to wash your hands!	☐	☐	☐

Calculation

Total Possible Points: _____

Total Points Earned: _____ Multiplied by 100 = _____ Divided by Total Possible Points = _____ %

Pass   Fail   Comments:

☐   ☐

Student's signature _____ Date _____

Partner's signature _____ Date _____

Instructor's signature _____ Date _____

Chapter 5

URINALYSIS

Chapter Competencies

Review the information in your textbook that supports the following course objectives.

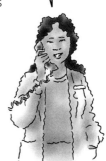

Make sure you have at least one classmate's e-mail address or phone number so you can get in touch if you have any questions.

Learning Objectives

- Explain why urinalysis is done and summarize the medical assistant's involvement in this process
- Describe the methods of urine collection
- Obtain a clean-catch midstream urine specimen
- Explain how and why urine specimens are tested
- Perform a chemical reagent test strip analysis
- Explain what a urine culture is and why it is done
- Identify the physical properties of urine and note some conditions that can affect them
- Determine the color and clarity of urine
- List the main chemical substances that may be found in urine and explain what the presence of each might mean
- Perform a Clinitest
- Perform a nitroprusside reaction (ACETEST) for ketones
- Perform an acid precipitation test for proteins
- Perform the diazo tablet test Ictotest (Ictotest) for bilirubin
- Identify substances that might be found in urine sediment and describe how urine sediment is examined
- Prepare urine sediment
- Describe how urine pregnancy tests are conducted
- Describe how urine drug tests are conducted

Learning Self-Assessment Exercises

KEY TERMS

Take advantage of your teacher's office hours to go over any confusing material.

Use the clues to unscramble the following terms. Copy the letters in the numbered cells to find the hidden message at the end of the puzzle.

RUCLETU a test in which bacteria and other microbes are grown in a lab to detect microorganisms causing a disease

☐☐☐☐☐☐☐
14

CIITERDUS drugs that increase the body's urine production

☐☐☐☐☐☐☐☐☐
3

TEUIHMAAR a condition in which blood is found in the urine

☐☐☐☐☐☐☐☐☐
5

AMEID a substance containing things bacteria need to grow

☐☐☐☐☐
15

TRUBDI urine that is cloudy

☐☐☐☐☐☐
2

LTPEICAATUR REAMTT tiny, solid particles that can be found in urine

☐☐☐☐☐☐☐☐☐☐☐
11

☐☐☐☐☐☐

SESTAPHOHP compounds made of phosphorous and oxygen

☐☐☐☐☐☐☐☐☐☐
8

TESARU nitrogen compounds produced when the body burns protein

☐☐☐☐☐☐
10

CIOGUSYRLA glucose in the urine

☐☐☐☐☐☐☐☐☐☐
17 6

GYIHYLMRPAECE high blood sugar

☐☐☐☐☐☐☐☐☐☐☐☐☐
7

LOITASCUGRAA high levels of galactose in urine and blood

☐☐☐☐☐☐☐☐☐☐☐☐
13

SOUTNREIRIPSD a nitrogen-cyanic compound that reacts with ketones to detect their presence in urine

☐☐☐☐☐☐☐☐☐☐☐☐☐
4

SMIENEDT solid matter that settles to the bottom of a liquid

☐☐☐☐☐☐☐☐
9

NARTESNUPAT the top liquid portion of spun urine

☐☐☐☐☐☐☐☐☐☐☐
1   16

SYLE to cause disintegration (i.e., destruction of adhesions, or the breakdown of red blood cells)

☐☐☐☐
12

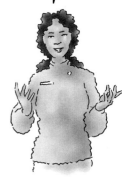

☐☐☐☐☐☐☐☐☐☐   ☐☐☐☐☐☐☐
1 2 3 4 5 6 7 8 9 10   11 12 13 14 15 16 17

PROCEDURE PRACTICE

Performing a Chemical Reagent Strip Analysis

Below is a sequence chart for performing a chemical reagent strip analysis. Fill in the missing steps with the choices from the answer bank on the next page.

1. Wash your hands.

↓

2. Assemble the equipment.

↓

3. _____

_____

↓

4. _____

_____

↓

5. Mix the patient's urine by gently swirling the specimen container. Then pour 12 mL of urine into a Kova system urine tube.

↓

6. _____

↓

7. Immerse the reagent strip in the urine completely, then immediately remove it, sliding the edge of the strip along the lip of the tube to remove excess urine. Turn the strip on its edge and touch the edge to a paper towel or other absorbent paper.

↓

8. _____

_____

↓

9. Compare the reagent pads to the color chart. Determine the results at intervals stated by the test strip manufacturer.

↓

10. _____

↓

11. _____

_____

↓

12. Properly care for or dispose of equipment and supplies. Clean the work area using a ten-percent bleach solution. Remove your gown, face shield, and gloves. Then, wash your hands.

ANSWER BANK

➤ Discard the used strip in a biohazard container. Discard the urine in accordance with your office's policies.

➤ Remove a reagent strip from its container and replace the lid to prevent deterioration of the strips by humidity. Do not remove the desiccant package from the container. It keeps moisture levels in the container to a minimum.

➤ Verify that the names on the specimen container and the report form are the same.

➤ Put on an impervious gown, a face shield, and gloves.

➤ Start your stopwatch or timer immediately after removing the strip from the urine. Reactions must be read at specific times as directed in the package insert and on the color comparison chart.

➤ Read all the reactions at the times indicated and record the results.

Labeling

The table shows the Normal Range for Physical Properties of Urine. Fill in the expected range for each property.

Normal Range for Physical Properties of Urine	
Property	**Expected Range**
Color	
Clarity	
Odor	
Specific gravity	

> It's great to form a study group, but it's best to keep the group between three and five people. If you have too many in your group, there's a greater chance of distractions.

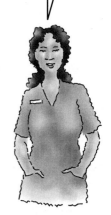

PRACTICE QUIZ

1. What is the type of urine collection in which a thin, sterile tube is inserted into the bladder through the urethra?
   a. bladder catheterization
   b. clean-catch method
   c. collection device
   d. suprapubic aspiration

2. The most concentrated urine is voided:
   a. before going to bed.
   b. after a person wakes up.
   c. after exercising for at least 20 minutes.
   d. All urine concentration is the same.

3. A patient provides a urine sample that is dark yellow. The color could indicate:
   a. the patient has hypertension.
   b. the patient has blood in the urine.
   c. the patient is dehydrated.
   d. the patient has too much fluid in his or her body tissues.

4. Why would a urine specimen need to be cultured?
   a. to find the urine's acidity
   b. to determine why there is blood in the urine
   c. to make sure there is not too much glucose in the urine
   d. to identify the bacteria causing a urinary tract infection

5. What would happen to the glucose in a person whose blood glucose level was higher than 180 mg/dL?
   a. It could pass out of the kidney into the urine
   b. It would reach the renal blood glucose threshold level.
   c. It would be broken down quickly in the body for energy.
   d. It would be stored in the kidney until the blood could absorb it.

6. Why should a urine sample be refrigerated if the testing is not going to be carried out for three hours?
   a. Refrigeration speeds up the changes in urine making it more acidic.
   b. Refrigeration slows down the growth of microorganisms.
   c. Refrigeration slows down the production of glucose in the urine.
   d. Refrigeration freezes the glucose in the urine so it can be scooped out.

7. Chemicals produced in the body when fat is metabolized are called:
   a. acetones.
   b. ketones.
   c. lipids.
   d. proteins.

8. Which of the following steps could cause the results of a clean-catch midstream urine specimen to be incorrect?
   a. Voiding for a second before collecting the sample.
   b. Using the antiseptic wipes provided before urinating.
   c. Using a new, clean, sterile container to collect the specimen.
   d. Placing the lid of the container in your pocket or bag so you don't contaminate it.

9. Which of the following statements about drug testing is NOT TRUE?
   a. Marijuana can't be detected in the urine.
   b. If an employer is paying for the test, he will receive all the results of the drug screening.
   c. The lab must use a commercial drug test approved by the U.S. Food and Drug Administration.
   d. If a drug is present in the urine, but its concentration is below the level required for a positive result, the overall outcome is negative.

10. Which of the following is not a physical property of urine?
    a. appearance
    b. color
    c. texture
    d. odor

CRITICAL THINKING PRACTICE

Conducting Lab Tests

1. A coworker is getting ready to perform a Clinitest on a patient's urine. When she gathers her equipment, she picks up plastic test tubes instead of glass test tubes. Explain to her why plastic test tubes can't be used.

   _____

   _____

   _____

   _____

2. You forget to set the timer while performing a chemical reagent strip analysis test. Explain how this could affect the results of the test.

_____

_____

_____

_____

Keep up with your work and reading throughout the class. This should make cramming for tests unnecessary.

3. You need to train a new medical assistant on how to prepare a urine sediment specimen. Explain why the urine specimen must be centrifuged and how to make the microscopic slide.

_____

_____

_____

_____

Results of Urinalysis

Review the chart below. Then answer the questions below and on the next page regarding the color variations in urine samples and the possible diagnosis.

Common Causes of Color Variations in Urine

Color	Possible Causes
Yellow-brown or amber	Bilirubin in urine (as in jaundice)
Dark yellow	Concentrated urine, low fluid intake, dehydration, inability of kidney to dilute urine, fluorescein (intravenous dye), multivitamins, excessive carotene
Bright orange-red	Pyridium (urinary tract analgesic)
Red or reddish-brown	Hemoglobin pigments, pyrvinium pamoate (Povan) medication for intestinal worms, sulfonamides (sulfa-based antibiotics)
Green or blue	Artificial color in food or drugs
Blackish, grayish, smoky	Hemoglobin or remains of old red blood cells (indicating bleeding in upper urinary tract), chyle, prostatic fluid, yeasts, homogentisic acid

1. A patient has been vomiting and suffering from severe diarrhea for two days. She says she has no appetite and can't keep down food or liquids. Her urine sample is dark yellow. What could be the cause?

_____

_____

2. A patient comes in to provide a urine sample for a urine drug test. Her urine sample is green. Is this a sign that she tampered with the test results?

_____

_____

3. A patient's urine sample is amber colored. What could be the cause?

_____

_____

4. A patient is taking antibiotics. She comes in to provide a urine sample and the urine is reddish-brown. What might be the cause?

_____

_____

Certification Prep

1. What will increase in a urine specimen if it's allowed to sit at room temperature?
   a. viruses
   b. bacteria
   c. nitrates
   d. mucus

2. What urine elements deteriorate if not tested or refrigerated within one hour of collecting the sample?
   a. Microorganisms multiply, alter the pH, and decrease glucose present in the urine.
   b. Yeast that may be present multiplies by budding process.
   c. Protein breaks down, increasing the level of ketones.
   d. Red blood cells (RBCs) break down and may give a false-negative to the presence of blood in the urine.

3. Dark yellow or amber urine may be a result of what?
   a. leukocytosis
   b. dehydration
   c. turbidity
   d. nephrolithiasis

4. What is the instrument called that is used to measure the density of urine?
   a. gravitometer
   b. microscope
   c. Clinitest
   d. refractometer

5. Which of the following does NOT describe a possible appearance of urine?
   a. hazy
   b. pungent
   c. straw
   d. turbid

6. What is the best method to collect a urine sample to check for a urinary tract infection?
   a. 24-hour specimen
   b. first morning specimen
   c. clean-catch, midstream specimen
   d. random specimen

7. What is a lab test in which microorganisms are grown in a nutrient medium to be identified called?
   a. culture
   b. Clinitest
   c. reagent test
   d. ketone test

8. How can dehydration or diabetes mellitus affect a urinalysis?
   a. elevated urine pH
   b. increased specific gravity
   c. pale yellow color
   d. low specific gravity

9. What medical disorders may cause concentrated urine?
   a. pneumonia, sinus infection, otitis media
   b. nausea, vomiting, perspiration, diabetes
   c. hydrophobia, hydropsy
   d. hydromeiosis, Krabbe's disease

Name _____ Date _____ Time _____

Task: With a partner as the patient, give accurate and complete instruction on how to obtain a clean-catch midstream urine specimen.

Conditions: The student will perform this task under the conditions described in the Procedure Steps, below.

Equipment/Supplies: a clean, dry (or sterile) urine container labeled with the patient's name; antiseptic wipes; a bedpan or urinal (if necessary); and gloves (if you'll be assisting the patient).

Standards: The student will perform this skill with _____ % accuracy in a total of _____ minutes. *(Your instructor will tell you what the percentage and time limits will be before you begin.)*

Key: 4 = Satisfactory   0 = Unsatisfactory   NA = this step is not counted

Procedure Steps	Self	Partner	Instructor
1. Gather your equipment. To obtain a clean-catch midstream urine specimen, you'll need the following: a clean, dry (or sterile) urine container labeled with the patient's name; antiseptic wipes; a bedpan or urinal (if necessary); and gloves (if you'll be assisting the patient).	☐	☐	☐
2. Wash your hands. Put on gloves if you'll be assisting the patient.	☐	☐	☐
3. Greet and identify the patient. Explain the procedure. Ask for and answer any questions the patient may have.	☐	☐	☐
4. If the patient will perform the procedure, give the patient the proper supplies.	☐	☐	☐
5. Tell patients that they must follow the procedure exactly or the specimen may be contaminated and produce false test results. Also, keep in mind that many patients might not know what the meatus or glans labia are, so be sure to explain in your instructions if necessary.	☐	☐	☐

Continued on back

	Self	Partner	Instructor
6. Instruct male patients: • Wash your hands upon entering the bathroom. Remove the lid from the container and place the lid flat side down in the designated area. Be careful not to touch the inside of the lid. • If uncircumcised, retract the foreskin to expose the glans penis. Clean the meatus with an antiseptic wipe. Use a new wipe for each cleaning sweep. • Keep the foreskin retracted and void for a second into the toilet or urinal. It's important to do this first so the specimen will have the least contamination with the skin. • While maintaining a stream, bring the sterile container into the urine stream. Collect 30 to 100 mL. Do not touch the inside of the container with the penis. • Once a sufficient amount has been collected, finish voiding into the toilet or urinal. • Cap the specimen container and wash your hands. Bring the container to the designated area. Test, transfer, or store the container according to your office's policy.	☐	☐	☐
7. Instruct female patients: • Wash your hands upon entering the bathroom. Remove the lid from the container and place the lid flat side down in the designated area. Be careful not to touch the inside of the lid. • Kneel or squat over a toilet or bedpan. Spread the labia minora to expose the meatus. First, cleanse on each side of the meatus. Wipe from front to back, using a new wipe for each side. Then, using a new wipe, clean the meatus itself. Again, wipe from front to back. • Keeping the labia separated, initially void for a second into the toilet or bedpan. It's important to do this first so the specimen will have the least contamination with the skin. • While maintaining a stream, bring the sterile container into the stream and collect 30 to 100 mL.	☐	☐	☐

	Self	Partner	Instructor
• Once a sufficient amount has been collected, finish voiding into the toilet or bedpan. • Cap the specimen container and wash your hands. Bring the container to the designated area. Test, transfer, or store the container according to your office's policy.			
8. Use gloves when handling the specimen container returned by the patient. Then, clean the work area, remove your gloves, and wash your hands.	☐	☐	☐
9. Record the procedure.	☐	☐	☐

Calculation

Total Possible Points: _____

Total Points Earned: _____ Multiplied by 100 = _____ Divided by Total Possible Points = _____ %

Pass   Fail   Comments:

☐   ☐

Student's signature _____ Date _____

Partner's signature _____ Date _____

Instructor's signature _____ Date _____

Hands On Procedure 5-2: Performing a Chemical Strip Analysis

Task: Perform a chemical strip analysis.

Conditions: The student will perform this task under the conditions described in the Procedure Steps, below.

Equipment/Supplies: a chemical strip (such as Multistix or Chemstrip); the manufacturer's color comparison chart; a stopwatch or timer; a 15 × 125 mm test tube or Kova system urine tube; a patient report form or data form

Standards: The student will perform this skill with _____ % accuracy in a total of _____ minutes. *(Your instructor will tell you what the percentage and time limits will be before you begin.)*

Key: 4 = Satisfactory   0 = Unsatisfactory   NA = this step is not counted

Procedure Steps	Self	Partner	Instructor
1. Wash your hands.	☐	☐	☐
2. Assemble the equipment: a chemical strip (such as Multistix or Chemstrip), the manufacturer's color comparision chart, a stopwatch or timer, a 15 × 125 mm test tube or Kova system urine tube, and a patient report form or data form.	☐	☐	☐
3. Put on an impervious gown, a face shield, and gloves.	☐	☐	☐
4. Verify that the names on the specimen container and the report form are the same.	☐	☐	☐
5. Mix the patient's urine by gently swirling the specimen container. Then pour 12 mL of urine into a Kova system urine tube.	☐	☐	☐
6. Remove a reagent strip from its container and replace the lid to prevent deterioration of the strips by humidity. Do not remove the desiccant package from the container. It keeps moisture levels in the container to a minimum.	☐	☐	☐

Continued on back

	Self	Partner	Instructor
7. Immerse the reagent strip in the urine completely, then immediately remove it, sliding the edge of the strip along the lip of the tube to remove excess urine. Turn the strip on its edge and touch the edge to a paper towel or other absorbent paper. Immediate removal and touching its edge to a paper towel prevents colors from leaching due to prolonged exposure to urine.	☐	☐	☐
8. Start your stopwatch or timer immediately after removing the strip from the urine. Reactions must be read at specific times as directed in the package insert and on the color comparison chart.	☐	☐	☐
9. Compare the reagent pads to the color chart. Determine the results at intervals stated by the test strip manufacturer. • Example: Glucose is read at 30 seconds. For that result, examine the glucose pad 30 seconds after dipping and compare it with the color chart for glucose.	☐	☐	☐
10. Read all the reactions at the times indicated and record the results.	☐	☐	☐
11. Discard the used strip in a biohazard container. Discard the urine in accordance with your office's policies.	☐	☐	☐
12. Properly care for or dispose of equipment and supplies. Clean the work area using a ten-percent bleach solution. Remove your gown, face shield, and gloves. Then, wash your hands.	☐	☐	☐

Calculation

Total Possible Points: _____

Total Points Earned: _____ Multiplied by 100 = _____ Divided by Total Possible Points = _____ %

Pass   Fail   Comments:

☐   ☐

Student's signature _____ Date _____

Partner's signature _____ Date _____

Instructor's signature _____ Date _____

Name _____ Date _____ Time _____

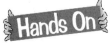 **Procedure 5-3:** Determining the Color
and Clarity of Urine

Task: Demonstrate how to properly determine the color and clarity of urine.

Conditions: The student will perform this task under the conditions described in the Procedure Steps, below.

Equipment/Supplies: a clear test tube; a sheet of white paper with scored black lines; a patient report form or data form

Standards: The student will perform this skill with _____ % accuracy in a total of _____ minutes. *(Your instructor will tell you what the percentage and time limits will be before you begin.)*

Key: 4 = Satisfactory   0 = Unsatisfactory   NA = this step is not counted

Procedure Steps	Self	Partner	Instructor
1. Wash your hands.	☐	☐	☐
2. Assemble the equipment: a clear test tube, a sheet of white paper with scored black lines, and a patient report form or data form.	☐	☐	☐
3. Put on gloves, an impervious gown, and a face shield.	☐	☐	☐
4. Verify that the names on the specimen container and the report form are the same.	☐	☐	☐
5. Pour 10 to 15 mL of urine from the container into the test tube.	☐	☐	☐
6. In a bright light against a white background, examine the color of the urine in the tube. • The intensity of yellow color, which is due to urochrome, depends on urine concentration. • The most common colors are straw (very pale yellow), yellow, and dark yellow.	☐	☐	☐

Continued on back

	Self	Partner	Instructor
7. Determine clarity by holding the tube in front of the white paper scored with black lines. • If you can see the lines clearly, record the sample as clear. • If the lines are not well defined when viewed through the sample, record it as hazy. • If you can't see the lines at all through the sample, record it as cloudy.	☐	☐	☐
8. If further testing is to be done but will be delayed more than an hour, refrigerate the specimen to avoid chemical changes.	☐	☐	☐
9. Properly care for or dispose of equipment and supplies. Clean the work area using a ten-percent bleach solution. Remove your gown, face shield, and gloves. Then, wash your hands.	☐	☐	☐

Calculation

Total Possible Points: _____

Total Points Earned: _____ Multiplied by 100 = _____ Divided by Total Possible Points = _____ %

Pass   Fail   Comments:

☐   ☐

Student's signature _____ Date _____

Partner's signature _____ Date _____

Instructor's signature _____ Date _____

Name _____ Date _____ Time _____

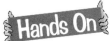 **Procedure 5-4:** Performing a Clinitest
for Reducing Sugars

Task: Perform a clinitest for reducing sugars.

Conditions: The student will perform this task under the conditions described in the Procedure Steps, below.

Equipment/Supplies: transfer pipettes; distilled water; positive and negative controls; a stopwatch or timer; a Clinitest color comparison chart; Clinitest tablets; a daily sample log; 16 × 125 mm glass test tubes; a test tube rack; a patient report form or data form

Standards: The student will perform this skill with _____ % accuracy in a total of _____ minutes. *(Your instructor will tell you what the percentage and time limits will be before you begin.)*

Key: 4 = Satisfactory   0 = Unsatisfactory   NA = this step is not counted

Procedure Steps	Self	Partner	Instructor
1. Wash your hands.	☐	☐	☐
2. Assemble the equipment: transfer pipettes, distilled water, positive and negative controls, a stopwatch or timer, a Clinitest color comparison chart, Clinitest tablets, a daily sample log, 16 × 125 mm glass test tubes, a test tube rack, and a patient report form or data form.	☐	☐	☐
3. Put on an impervious gown, a face shield, and gloves.	☐	☐	☐
4. Identify the specimen to be tested and record patient and sample information in the daily log.	☐	☐	☐
5. Record on the report or data form the patient's identification information, catalog and lot numbers for all test and control materials, and expiration dates. This is required by CLIA regulations and QA/QC procedures.	☐	☐	☐
6. Label test tubes with patient and control identification and put them in the test tube rack.	☐	☐	☐

Continued on back

	Self	Partner	Instructor
7. Using a transfer pipette, add ten drops of distilled water to each labeled test tube in the rack. Hold the dropper vertically to ensure proper delivery of the drops into the tube.	☐	☐	☐
8. Add five drops of the patient's urine or five drops of control sample to each tube, according to its label (for example, positive control sample to the tube labeled *positive control* and so on). Use a different transfer pipette for each tube. This prevents contaminating any of the samples.	☐	☐	☐
9. Open the Clinitest bottle and shake a tablet into the lid without touching it. Then drop the tablet from the lid into the test tube. Repeat for all patient and control samples being tested. Close the Clinitest bottle. • Touching the tablet may cause false results. • The Clinitest bottle must be kept tightly capped at all times because moisture causes the tablets to deteriorate. This will affect test results.	☐	☐	☐
10. Observe reactions in the test tubes as the mixture boils. After the reaction stops, wait 15 seconds, then gently swirl the test tubes. This mixes the contents so you can read the results. • Watch carefully during the boiling to see if the contents of the patient's tube pass through all the colors on the five-drop color chart before ending in a final color. • If this happens, the test result should be reported as "exceeds 2%." • If your lab requires a more exact result on this pass-through reaction, perform the two-drop method according to the Clinitest package insert and use the two-drop color chart for interpretation.	☐	☐	☐

	Self	Partner	Instructor
11. Immediately compare results for the patient specimen and the controls with the five-drop method color chart. • The positive and negative controls ensure testing accuracy. • If the positive and negative controls do not give expected results, the test is invalid and must be repeated. • Certain medications (for example, ascorbic acid) and reducing substances other than glucose (galactose and lactose) may cause false-positive results. If this occurs, further testing is necessary.	☐	☐	☐
12. Properly care for or dispose of equipment and supplies. Clean the work area using a ten-percent bleach solution. Remove your gown, face shield, and gloves. Then, wash your hands.	☐	☐	☐

Calculation

Total Possible Points: _____

Total Points Earned: _____ Multiplied by 100 = _____ Divided by Total Possible Points = _____ %

Pass ☐   Fail ☐   Comments:

Student's signature _____ Date _____

Partner's signature _____ Date _____

Instructor's signature _____ Date _____

Name _____ Date _____ Time _____

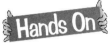 **Procedure 5-5:** Performing a Nitroprusside Reaction (ACETEST) for Ketones

Task: Perform a nitroprusside reaction (ACETEST) for ketones.

Conditions: The student will perform this task under the conditions described in the Procedure Steps, below.

Equipment/Supplies: white filter paper; a plastic transfer pipette; an ACETEST tablet; the manufacturer's color comparison chart; a stopwatch or timer that displays time to the second; a patient report form or data form

Standards: The student will perform this skill with _____ % accuracy in a total of _____ minutes. *(Your instructor will tell you what the percentage and time limits will be before you begin.)*

Key: 4 = Satisfactory   0 = Unsatisfactory   NA = this step is not counted

Procedure Steps	Self	Partner	Instructor
1. Wash your hands.	☐	☐	☐
2. Assemble the equipment: white filter paper, a plastic transfer pipette, an ACETEST tablet, the manufacturer's color comparison chart, a stopwatch or timer that displays time to the second, and a patient report form or data form.	☐	☐	☐
3. Put on an impervious gown, a face shield, and gloves.	☐	☐	☐
4. Identify the specimen to be tested and record patient and sample information in the daily log.	☐	☐	☐
5. Record on the report or data form the patient's identification information, catalog and lot numbers for all test and control materials, and expiration dates. This is required by CLIA regulations and QA/QC procedures.	☐	☐	☐

Continued on back

	Self	Partner	Instructor

6. Shake an ACETEST tablet into the cap and put it on the filter paper. Replace the cap.
  • Dispensing the tablet in this manner prevents contamination of the tablet or the bottle's contents.
  • The white background of the filter paper provides contrast for the test results.
	☐	☐	☐

7. Using a transfer pipette, place one drop of urine on top of the tablet.	☐	☐	☐
8. Wait 30 seconds for the complete reaction. A reaction will occur if ketones are present in the urine.	☐	☐	☐
9. Compare the color of the tablet to the manufacturer's color chart. Record the results as negative, small amount, moderate amount, or large amount.	☐	☐	☐
10. Properly care for or dispose of equipment and supplies. Clean the work area using a ten-percent bleach solution. Remove your gown, face shield, and gloves. Then, wash your hands.	☐	☐	☐

Calculation

Total Possible Points: _____

Total Points Earned: _____ Multiplied by 100 = _____ Divided by Total Possible Points = _____ %

Pass   Fail   Comments:
☐   ☐

Student's signature _____ Date _____

Partner's signature _____ Date _____

Instructor's signature _____ Date _____

Name _____ Date _____ Time _____

Procedure 5-6: Performing an Acid Precipitation Test for Protein

Task: Perform an acid precipitation test for protein.

Conditions: The student will perform this task under the conditions described in the Procedure Steps, below.

Equipment/Supplies: a test tube rack; clear test tubes; transfer pipettes; positive and negative controls; a stopwatch or timer; a daily sample log; three-percent sulfosalicylic acid (SSA) solution; a patient report form or data form

Standards: The student will perform this skill with _____ % accuracy in a total of _____ minutes. *(Your instructor will tell you what the percentage and time limits will be before you begin.)*

Key: 4 = Satisfactory   0 = Unsatisfactory   NA = this step is not counted

Procedure Steps	Self	Partner	Instructor
1. Wash your hands.	☐	☐	☐
2. Assemble the equipment: a test tube rack, clear test tubes, transfer pipettes, positive and negative controls, a stopwatch or timer, a daily sample log, three-percent sulfosalicylic acid (SSA) solution, and a patient report form or data form.	☐	☐	☐
3. Put on an impervious gown, a face shield, and gloves.	☐	☐	☐
4. Identify the patient's specimen to be tested and record patient and sample information on the daily log. This step prevents errors and fulfills QA/QC requirements.	☐	☐	☐
5. Record on the report or data form the patient's name or identification, catalog and lot numbers for all test and control materials, and expiration dates. This step fulfills QA/QC requirements.	☐	☐	☐
6. Label the test tubes with patient and control identification. Then place them in the test tube rack.	☐	☐	☐

Continued on back

	Self	Partner	Instructor
7. Centrifuge the patient sample at 1,500 rpm for five minutes.	☐	☐	☐
8. Add 1 to 3 mL of supernatant urine or control sample to the patient and control-labeled tubes in the rack. Use a clean transfer pipette for each.	☐	☐	☐
9. Add an equal amount of three-percent SSA to the sample quantity in each tube.	☐	☐	☐
10. Mix the contents of the tubes and let them stand for two to ten minutes. Use a stopwatch or timer to make sure you perform the next step within this time frame.	☐	☐	☐
11. Mix the contents of the tubes again, then observe the degree of turbidity in each test tube. Assign a score according to the following guidelines. • Neg: no turbidity or cloudiness; urine remains clear • Trace: slight turbidity • 1+: turbidity with no precipitation • 2+: heavy turbidity with fine granulation • 3+: heavy turbidity with granulation and flakes • 4+: clumps of precipitated protein	☐	☐	☐
12. The specimen may be matched against a McFarland standard for objective assessment. If positive and negative controls don't give the expected results, the test is invalid and must be repeated.	☐	☐	☐
13. Properly care for or dispose of equipment and supplies. Clean the work area using a ten-percent bleach solution. Remove your gown, face shield, and gloves. Then, wash your hands.	☐	☐	☐

Calculation

Total Possible Points: _____

Total Points Earned: _____ Multiplied by 100 = _____ Divided by Total Possible Points = _____ %

Pass   Fail   Comments:

☐   ☐

Student's signature _____ Date _____

Partner's signature _____ Date _____

Instructor's signature _____ Date _____

Hands On · Procedure 5-7: Performing the Diazo Tablet Test (Ictotest) for Bilirubin

Task: Perform the diazo tablet test (Ictotest) for bilirubin.

Conditions: The student will perform this task under the conditions described in the Procedure Steps, below.

Equipment/Supplies: Ictotest white mats; a stopwatch or timer; a transfer pipette; diazo (Ictotest) tablets; a clean paper towel; a patient report form or data form.

Standards: The student will perform this skill with _____ % accuracy in a total of _____ minutes. *(Your instructor will tell you what the percentage and time limits will be before you begin.)*

Key: 4 = Satisfactory   0 = Unsatisfactory   NA = this step is not counted

Procedure Steps	Self	Partner	Instructor
1. Wash your hands.	☐	☐	☐
2. Assemble the equipment: Ictotest white mats, a stopwatch or timer, a transfer pipette, diazo (Ictotest) tablets, a clean paper towel, and a patient report form or data form.	☐	☐	☐
3. Put on an impervious gown, a face shield, and gloves.	☐	☐	☐
4. Verify that the names on the specimen container and the report form are the same.	☐	☐	☐
5. Place the Ictotest white mat on a clean, dry paper towel. • The mat provides a testing surface. • The paper towel must be dry because moisture may cause a false result.	☐	☐	☐
6. Using a clean transfer pipette, add ten drops of urine to the center of the mat. • If the urine is red, it may be difficult to read the reaction properly. In this case, pour an aliquot of the urine into a urine tube or test tube.	☐	☐	☐

Continued on back

	Self	Partner	Instructor
• Centrifuge as if preparing urine sediment. (See the following Hands On Procedure.) Use ten drops of the supernatant in this step.			
7. Shake a diazo tablet into the bottle cap and put it into the center of the mat. Do not touch the tablet. Touching it contaminates it and could cause a false-positive result.	☐	☐	☐
8. Recap the bottle immediately to prevent the other tablets from deteriorating. The tablets must be protected from exposure to light, heat, and moisture.	☐	☐	☐
9. Use a clean transfer pipette to place one drop of water on the tablet. Then wait five seconds.	☐	☐	☐
10. Add another drop of water to the tablet so that the solution formed by the first drop runs onto the mat. This lets the diazo chemical react with the urine.	☐	☐	☐
11. Within 60 seconds, observe for color on the mat around the tablet. • A blue or purple color indicates a positive result for bilirubin. • A pink or red color indicates a negative result.	☐	☐	☐
12. Properly care for or dispose of equipment and supplies. Clean the work area using a ten-percent bleach solution. Remove your gown, face shield, and gloves. Then, wash your hands.	☐	☐	☐

Calculation

Total Possible Points: _____

Total Points Earned: _____ Multiplied by 100 = _____ Divided by Total Possible Points = _____ %

Pass   Fail   Comments:
☐   ☐

Student's signature _____ Date _____

Partner's signature _____ Date _____

Instructor's signature _____ Date _____

Hands On — **Procedure 5-8:** Preparing Urine Sediment

Task: Prepare urine sediment.

Conditions: The student will perform this task under the conditions described in the Procedure Steps, below.

Equipment/Supplies: a centrifuge; urine centrifuge tubes; a transfer pipette; a patient report form or data form.

Standards: The student will perform this skill with _____ % accuracy in a total of _____ minutes. *(Your instructor will tell you what the percentage and time limits will be before you begin.)*

Key: 4 = Satisfactory   0 = Unsatisfactory   NA = this step is not counted

Procedure Steps	Self	Partner	Instructor
1. Wash your hands.	☐	☐	☐
2. Assemble the equipment: a centrifuge, urine centrifuge tubes, a transfer pipette, and a patient report form or data form.	☐	☐	☐
3. Put on an impervious gown, a face shield, and gloves.	☐	☐	☐
4. Verify that the names on the specimen container and the report form are the same.	☐	☐	☐
5. Swirl the specimen to mix. Pour 10 to 12 mL of well-mixed urine into a labeled urine centrifuge tube or a tube provided by the test system manufacturer. Cap the tube with a plastic cap or parafilm. • Some test systems use 10 mL and some use 12 mL. The 12 mL volume allows reagent strip testing from the same tube. Check your lab procedures to find out which type of tube to use. • Some patients can't produce a large amount of urine. If less than the standard 10 or 12 mL of urine is available, document the actual volume prepared on the report form. This is necessary to ensure proper interpretation of results.	☐	☐	☐

Continued on back

	Self	Partner	Instructor
• Preparing a urine sediment sample from less than three mL of specimen is not recommended.			
6. Centrifuge the sample at 1,500 rpm for five minutes. This ensures that cellular and particulate matter is pulled to the bottom of the tube.	☐	☐	☐
7. When the centrifuge has stopped, remove the tubes. After making sure that no tests are to be performed first on the supernatant, pour off all but 0.5 to 1.0 mL of it. Follow the manufacturer's directions for this procedure.	☐	☐	☐
8. Suspend the sediment again in the remaining supernatant by aspirating up into the bulbous portion of a urine transfer pipette.	☐	☐	☐
9. Place a urine slide (kova slide or other urine system slide) on the counter. Add a drop of the mixed sediment on the slide with built-in coverslip. (Follow the test system's manufacturer's directions for doing this.) The concentrated urine is now prepared for microscopic examination.	☐	☐	☐
10. Properly care for or dispose of equipment and supplies. Clean the work area using a ten-percent bleach solution. Remove your gown, face shield, and gloves. Then, wash your hands.	☐	☐	☐

Calculation

Total Possible Points: _____

Total Points Earned: _____ Multiplied by 100 = _____ Divided by Total Possible Points = _____ %

Pass   Fail   Comments:

☐   ☐

Student's signature _____ Date _____

Partner's signature _____ Date _____

Instructor's signature _____ Date _____

Chapter 6

CLINICAL CHEMISTRY

Chapter Competencies

Review the information in your textbook that supports the following course objectives.

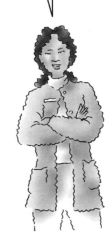

Schedule your study time for the time of day when you're most alert instead of squeezing it in at the end of the day.

Learning Objectives

- Explain the purpose of performing clinical chemistry tests
- List the common panels of chemistry tests
- List the instruments used for chemical testing
- List tests used to evaluate renal function
- List the common electrolytes and explain the relationship of electrolytes to body function
- Describe the nonprotein nitrogenous compounds and name conditions associated with abnormal values
- Describe the substances commonly tested in liver function assessment
- Explain thyroid function and identify the hormone that regulates the thyroid gland
- Describe how laboratory tests help assess for a myocardial infarction
- Describe how pancreatitis is diagnosed with laboratory tests
- Explain how the body uses and regulates glucose and summarize the purpose of the major glucose tests
- Determine a patient's blood glucose level
- Perform glucose tolerance testing
- Describe the function of cholesterol and other lipids and their correlation to heart disease

Learning Self-Assessment Exercises

KEY TERMS

Complete the word search puzzle below with the appropriate key terms. Words may be backward and diagonal, and letters may be used for more than one clue. (Hint: It may be helpful to determine which words you are seeking before searching the puzzle.) Refer to the list of clues at right.

```
W C A A E Z A F Q A P O X D I
T R J V N R L J T T E D Z O C
Y E W W H I S P A H D Q N S T
X A E L I B O Q W E C S C U S
A T U Y U E Q N S R S Y V O S
S I S O D I C A S O C Y R N X
E N D O C R I N E S Y S T E M
N E T A N O B R A C I B E G Q
E G L U C A G O N L J R D O P
G I S O E N Z Y M E T W E R W
O U O D T F F T K R Z D M T N
C T F X J J H Z G O M Q A I C
Y P L I V K F H D S H O P N N
L F U D I T N H F I N C A W A
G M K C J P Z B R S K R U J W
```

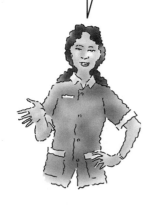

Keeping all of your notes and class information in one notebook, folder, or binder will help you stay organized and make study time easier.

1. a negatively charged ion
2. a chemical compound in the body that adds phosphorus to ADP to make ATP, which is the energy currency in the body
3. the body system made up of hormones and the glands that secrete them
4. a condition of excess acid in the body fluids
5. buildup of fatty plaque on the interior lining of arteries causing the arteries to narrow and harden
6. any enzyme or group of enzymes that have the same functions in the body but different physical and chemical makeups
7. electrically charged atoms
8. swelling due to excess fluid
9. dissolved carbon dioxide
10. bitter, yellow-green secretion of the liver that is stored in the gallbladder
11. relating to or containing nitrogen
12. the stored form of glucose
13. the hormone that stimulates the release of glycogen

PROCEDURE PRACTICE

Determining Blood Glucose

Below is a sequence for determining blood glucose. The sequence is in the incorrect order. Next to each number, fill in the letter that coincides with that step in the sequence. Steps 1 and 2 have been completed for you.

A. Gather your equipment and supplies.

B. Wash your hands and put on your gloves before you remove the reagent strip from the container.

C. Cleanse the puncture site (finger) with alcohol.

D. Remove one reagent strip, lay it on the paper towel, and recap the container.

E. Bring the reagent strip up to the finger and touch the strip to the blood. Make sure you don't touch the finger. Then insert the reagent strip into the glucose meter.

F. Turn on the glucose meter and make sure that it's calibrated correctly. Otherwise, the test results may be inaccurate.

G. Care for and dispose of your equipment and supplies. Clean your work area. Then, remove your gloves and wash your hands.

1. A
2. B
3. _____
4. _____
5. _____
6. _____
7. _____
8. _____
9. _____
10. _____
11. _____
12. _____
13. _____

(*continued on next page*)

H. Greet and identify the patient. Explain the procedure and ask for and answer any questions the patient might have. Ask the patient when she last ate and document this in her chart.

I. The instrument reads the reaction strip and displays the result on the screen in milligrams per deciliter (mg/dL). If the glucose level is higher or lower than expected, review the troubleshooting guide provided by the manufacturer.

J. Turn the patient's hand palm down and gently squeeze the finger so that a large drop of blood forms. You must squeeze gently to avoid diluting the sample with tissue fluid.

K. Apply a small adhesive bandage to the patient's fingertip.

L. Apply pressure to the puncture wound with gauze. While you are doing this, the meter will incubate the strip and measure the reaction.

M. Perform a capillary puncture. Wipe away the first drop of blood.

Understanding Electrolytes

Electrolytes are ions in the blood and body fluids. The following table shows the most common electrolytes found in the blood. Fill in the missing spaces in the table.

Common Electrolytes Found in the Blood

Electrolyte	Anion or Cation	Symbol	Normal Serum Levels mEq/L
Sodium	_____	_____	135 to 145 mEq/L
_____	_____	K	3.5 to 5.0 mEq/L
Chloride	_____	_____	_____
Calcium	Cation	_____	_____
Magnesium	_____	_____	1.3 to 2.1 mEq/L
_____	_____	P	_____
Bicarbonate	_____	_____	22 to 29 mmoles/L of total CO_2

PRACTICE QUIZ

1. How can a patient develop edema?
   a. Edema develops when there is too much carbon dioxide in the blood.
   b. Edema develops when there are more anions in the blood than cations.
   c. Edema develops when arteries get clogged with a buildup of fatty plaque.
   d. Edema develops when the kidneys begin to fail and waste products build up in the blood.

2. Why is it important for a physician to know the amount of chemical substances in the body?
   a. It helps the physician check the function of certain organs.
   b. It helps the physician make sure there are no ions in the body.
   c. It helps the physician calculate the blood volume of a patient.
   d. It helps the physician determine if the body is producing antibodies when exposed to a disease.

3. The type of glucose test in which blood can be drawn at any time is called a:
   a. glucose tolerance test.
   b. fasting blood sugar.
   c. random blood glucose.
   d. two-hour postprandial glucose.

4. How is cholesterol beneficial to the body?
   a. It helps remove wastes from the blood.
   b. It helps insulin to move out of the blood into the cells.
   c. It helps form bile acids that are produced in the liver and stored in the gallbladder.
   d. It is not beneficial to the body because it leads to the development of atherosclerosis.

5. Which condition can be determined by a fasting glucose level?
   a. atherosclerosis
   b. diabetes
   c. hypertension
   d. pancreatitis

6. Which items should be disposed of in the biohazard waste container?
   a. needles
   b. broken glass
   c. disposable tray wrappers
   d. soiled examination gloves

7. Measuring levels of urea in the blood can tell a physician how which of the following organs are functioning?
   a. heart and brain
   b. kidney and liver
   c. spleen and liver
   d. urinary bladder and large intestine

8. Which of the following is NOT an electrolyte found in the blood?
   a. calcium
   b. chloride
   c. glucose
   d. sodium

9. All of the following are benefits of using an automated system for chemical analysis except:
   a. fewer operator errors.
   b. employing more workers.
   c. less expensive testing costs.
   d. providing faster test results.

10. Elevated levels of bilirubin in a patient's blood can be a sign of disease in which of the following organs?
    a. heart
    b. kidney
    c. liver
    d. lungs

CRITICAL THINKING PRACTICE

Calculating a Patient's Cardiac Risk

To estimate a patient's cardiac risk, divide the patient's total cholesterol figure by his HDL figure.

- A result of four indicates normal cardiac risk.
- A number less than four indicates a decreased cardiac risk.
- A number higher than four indicates an increased cardiac risk.

Fill in the table below. First, find each patient's cardiac risk. Then, decide if the patient has a normal, decreased, or increased cardiac risk. The first one is filled in for you.

Arriving to class on time will help you to keep up with the work.

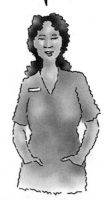

Examples of Cardiac Risk

Patient	Total Cholesterol (mg/dL)	HDL (mg/dL)	Result	Cardiac Risk
1	180	45	4	Normal
2	150	25	_____	_____
3	210	70	_____	_____
4	195	65	_____	_____
5	180	30	_____	_____
6	200	50	_____	_____

Insulin and Glucagon

Consider each scenario below. Then decide if blood glucose levels would rise
or decrease. As a result, when would insulin or glucagon need to be released
into the blood? First circle *Increase* or *Decrease* and then explain why.

1. A person has a high carbohydrate dinner.

   Increase   Decrease

   _____

   _____

2. A high school football player has just finished afternoon practice.

   Increase   Decrease

   _____

   _____

3. A person wakes up in the morning and eats breakfast.

   Increase   Decrease

   _____

   _____

4. A student wakes up in the morning, goes to class, and does not eat his first meal until 2:00 P.M.

   Increase   Decrease

   _____

   _____

Certification Prep

1. Which statement about high-density lipoprotein (HDL) is NOT accurate?
   a. HDL typically exists in lesser quantities than low-density lipoprotein (LDL).
   b. HDL is sometimes called "the good lipid."
   c. HDL's protein molecules carry cholesterol deposited on artery walls back to the liver.
   d. Little research has been directed along the lines of increasing HDL.

2. When the kidneys begin to fail, what happens?
   a. Emergency treatment is not necessary as the prognosis for recovery is very good.
   b. The patient loses weight because of increased loss of fluids.
   c. Waste products, such as urea, ammonia, and creatinine, build up in the blood.
   d. Serum measurements of lipids will be checked.

3. Which statement best explains why obstetric patients are sometimes asked to have a glucose tolerance test (GTT)?
   a. This screening method is usually done during the second trimester.
   b. A decrease of glucose intolerance has been frequently noted among pregnant patients.
   c. An increase of glucose intolerance has been frequently noted among pregnant patients.
   d. This screening method helps evaluate kidney function in a pregnant patient.

4. Which statement about chloride is accurate?
   a. Chloride supplements are available in enriched dairy products.
   b. In hyperchloremia, the serum chloride level is above 16 mEq/L.
   c. The normal range for chloride is 16 to 46 mEq/L.
   d. Chloride is the major anion of the extracellular fluid.

5. Which statement about electrolytes is NOT accurate?
   a. They aid in the functioning of nerve cells and muscle tissue.
   b. They are only positively charged.
   c. They are ions (chemicals that carry a charge) found in blood and body fluids.
   d. They help maintain fluid and acid-base balance.

6. How can quantifying amounts of metabolic by-products contained in body fluids assist the doctor?
   a. to assess organ function (e.g., bilirubin level is an indicator of liver function)
   b. to indicate whether or not to treat for lead poisoning
   c. to decide on a weight-loss program for the patient
   d. to indicate if a fluid restriction needs to be enforced

7. What statement below best defines troponin?
   a. A troponin sample is obtained with a green or yellow top serum tube.
   b. Troponin is a protein specific to heart muscle.
   c. Sometimes it is used to diagnose myocardial infarction.
   d. It is a test that is done by analyzing a blood serum sample.

8. Which statement about sodium is accurate?
   a. Normal serum levels range from 100 to 200 mEq/L.
   b. Hypernatremia is a sodium level above 100 mEq/L.
   c. Sodium (Na) is the major cation of the extracellular fluid (the fluid outside the cell).
   d. Hyponatremia is a sodium level below 200 mEq/L.

9. Which statement best explains the role of the thyroid gland?
   a. Situations can cause an imbalance in this delicate endocrine system.
   b. If the thyroid gland is malfunctioning, it cannot be stimulated.
   c. It is controlled by another hormone, TSH, produced in the anterior pituitary gland.
   d. Anterior pituitary gland malfunction may result in oversecretion/undersecretion of TSH.

10. Which statement about bicarbonate is NOT accurate?
    a. The acid-base system is extremely sensitive and cannot tolerate large pH fluctuations.
    b. Bicarbonate is formed when carbon dioxide dissolves in the bloodstream.
    c. Bicarbonate is the major factor in acid-base balance.
    d. Bicarbonate is breathed out in the form of chloride and also excreted through the kidneys.

Hands On Procedure 6-1: Determining Blood Glucose

Task: With a partner as the patient, obtain a blood sample using capillary puncture, then determine blood glucose.

Conditions: The student will perform this task under the conditions described in the Procedure Steps, below.

Equipment/Supplies: glucose meter; glucose reagent strips; a lancet; an alcohol pad; sterile gauze; a paper towel; an adhesive bandage; gloves

Standards: The student will perform this skill with ____ % accuracy in a total of ____ minutes. *(Your instructor will tell you what the percentage and time limits will be before you begin.)*

Key: 4 = Satisfactory 0 = Unsatisfactory NA = this step is not counted

Procedure Steps	Self	Partner	Instructor
1. Gather your equipment and supplies: a glucose meter of the physician's choice, glucose reagent strips, a lancet, an alcohol pad, sterile gauze, a paper towel, an adhesive bandage, and gloves.	☐	☐	☐
2. Wash your hands and put on your gloves before you remove the reagent strip from the container.	☐	☐	☐
3. Turn on the glucose meter and make sure that it's calibrated correctly. Otherwise, the test results may be inaccurate.	☐	☐	☐
4. Remove one reagent strip, lay it on the paper towel, and recap the container. The strip is ready for testing and the paper towel serves as a disposable work surface. It will also absorb any excess blood.	☐	☐	☐
5. Greet and identify the patient. Explain the procedure, and ask for and answer any questions the patient might have. Ask the patient when she last ate and document this in her chart.	☐	☐	☐
6. Cleanse the puncture site (finger) with alcohol.	☐	☐	☐
7. Perform a capillary puncture, following the steps outlined in Chapter 2. Wipe away the first drop of blood.	☐	☐	☐

Continued on back

	Self	Partner	Instructor
8. Turn the patient's hand palm down and gently squeeze the finger so that a large drop of blood forms. You must squeeze gently to avoid diluting the sample with tissue fluid.	☐	☐	☐
9. Bring the reagent strip up to the finger and touch the strip to the blood. Make sure you don't touch the finger. Then insert the reagent strip into the glucose meter.	☐	☐	☐
10. Apply pressure to the puncture wound with gauze. While you are doing this, the meter will incubate the strip and measure the reaction.	☐	☐	☐
11. The instrument reads the reaction strip and displays the result on the screen in milligrams per deciliter (mg/dL). If the glucose level is higher or lower than expected, review the troubleshooting guide provided by the manufacturer. Controls are available in the low, normal, and high range to ensure that the glucose meter is functioning properly. These controls should run daily according to the manufacturer's instructions.	☐	☐	☐
12. Apply a small adhesive bandage to the patient's fingertip.	☐	☐	☐
13. Care for and dispose of your equipment and supplies. Clean your work area. Then, remove your gloves and wash your hands.	☐	☐	☐

Calculation

Total Possible Points: _____

Total Points Earned: _____ Multiplied by 100 = _____ Divided by Total Possible Points = _____ %

Pass   Fail   Comments:

☐   ☐

Student's signature _____ Date _____

Partner's signature _____ Date _____

Instructor's signature _____ Date _____

Hands On Procedure 6-2: Glucose Tolerance Testing

Task: Demonstrate how to perform a 3-hour glucose tolerance test.

Conditions: The student will perform this task under the conditions described in the Procedure Steps, below.

Equipment/Supplies: calibrated amount of glucose solution per physician's order; glucose meter equipment; phlebotomy equipment; glucose test strips; alcohol wipes; a stopwatch; gloves

Standards: The student will perform this skill with _____ % accuracy in a total of _____ minutes. *(Your instructor will tell you what the percentage and time limits will be before you begin.)*

Key: 4 = Satisfactory   0 = Unsatisfactory   NA = this step is not counted

Procedure Steps	Self	Partner	Instructor
1. Gather the following equipment and supplies: calibrated amount of glucose solution per physician's order, glucose meter equipment, phlebotomy equipment, glucose test strips, alcohol wipes, a stopwatch, and gloves. The stopwatch is particularly important because the timing of the blood collections has a direct effect on test results.	☐	☐	☐
2. Greet and identify the patient. Explain the procedure, and ask for and answer any questions the patient might have. Ask the patient when he last ate and document this in his chart.	☐	☐	☐
3. Wash your hands and put on your gloves.	☐	☐	☐
4. Obtain a fasting glucose (FBS) specimen from the patient by venipuncture or capillary puncture as explained in Chapter 2. • It's recommended that a lab test the fasting blood sample before the patient ingests the glucose drink. • If the FBS exceeds 140 mg/dL, do not perform the test. Instead, inform the physician. • Giving more glucose to a patient whose blood glucose level is too high could seriously harm the patient.	☐	☐	☐

Continued on back

	Self	Partner	Instructor
5. Give the glucose drink to the patient, and ask the patient to drink it all within five minutes. The body starts to metabolize the glucose right away, so the patient must drink rapidly.	☐	☐	☐
6. Note the time the patient finishes the drink; this is the official start of the test. Keep the following things in mind during the test: • The patient should remain mostly inactive during this procedure because exercise alters the glucose levels by increasing the body's demand for energy. • The patient should not smoke during the test because smoking can artificially increase the glucose level. • The patient may drink water, but only water. • If the patient has any severe symptoms (for example, headache, dizziness, vomiting), obtain a blood specimen at that time. Then end the test and inform the physician. These symptoms could indicate intolerably high or low glucose levels.	☐	☐	☐
7. Obtain another blood specimen exactly 30 minutes after the patient finishes the glucose drink. Label the specimen with the patient's name and time of collection. Follow the precautions listed in step 6 for the remainder of the test. The physician may want urine glucose tests done with each blood sample taken. Ask the patient to submit a urine sample after you take the blood sample. Never attempt to get the urine sample before the blood sample as it might cause you to miss the timer for the blood sample. If the patient doesn't provide a urine sample, don't worry about it. Submit an empty urine cup in place of an actual urine sample and label "patient could not provide urine sample at ### time." Note: It is absolutely vital to the accuracy of the test that you are precise with the timing of the blood collections. Make all proper notations so the results can be accurately interpreted.	☐	☐	☐
8. Exactly one hour after the glucose drink, repeat step 7.	☐	☐	☐

	Self	Partner	Instructor
9. Exactly two hours after the glucose drink, repeat step 7.	☐	☐	☐
10. Exactly three hours after the glucose drink, repeat step 7. Unless a test longer than three hours has been ordered, the test is now complete. Otherwise, continue with the test for the specified period of time. Sometimes, the test can be up to six hours to detect hypoglycemia.	☐	☐	☐
11. If the specimens are going to be tested by an outside laboratory, package them carefully and arrange for transportation.	☐	☐	☐
12. Care for and dispose of your equipment and supplies. Clean your work area. Then, remove your gloves and wash your hands.	☐	☐	☐

Calculation

Total Possible Points: _____

Total Points Earned: _____ Multiplied by 100 = _____ Divided by Total Possible Points = _____ %

Pass   Fail   Comments:

☐   ☐

Student's signature _____ Date _____

Partner's signature _____ Date _____

Instructor's signature _____ Date _____

Chapter 7

MICROBIOLOGY

Chapter Competencies

Review the information in your textbook that supports the following course objectives.

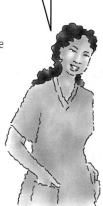

Reviewing your notes after class will help to reinforce the newly learned concepts.

Learning Objectives

- Describe how cultures are used in medical microbiology and explain what media and colonies are
- Name and describe the different types of bacteria
- Identify the main types of fungi that may be found in the human body
- Identify different types of viruses
- Identify the two main types of metazoa and give at least one example of each
- Summarize the medical assistant's responsibilities in microbiological testing
- List the most common microbiological specimens collected in the physician's office lab
- Collect a specimen for throat culture
- Collect a sputum specimen
- Collect a stool specimen
- Test a stool specimen for occult blood
- Explain how to transport a specimen
- State the difference between primary cultures, secondary cultures, and pure cultures
- Name at least three kinds of media used in cultures
- Explain how to care for media plates
- Summarize the ways of inoculating media
- Inoculate a culture using dilution streaking
- Inoculate for drug sensitivity testing using "even lawn" streaking
- Inoculate for quantitative culturing or urine colony count using "even lawn" streaking
- Describe how microscopic examination is used in medical microbiology
- Prepare a wet mount slide
- Prepare a dry smear
- State the purpose of Gram staining and summarize the process
- Gram stain a smear slide

Learning Self-Assessment Exercises

A study group provides an opportunity to share what you know and also learn from other group members.

KEY TERMS

Use the clues to unscramble each of the key terms. Copy the letters in the numbered cells to find the hidden message at the end of the puzzle.

GEASOTNHP disease-causing microorganisms

☐☐☐☐☐☐☐☐☐☐
                5

GOOVYRLI the study of viruses

☐☐☐☐☐☐☐☐☐
           10

DEMIA special material used when culturing specimens that helps bacteria present in the specimen to grow

☐☐☐☐☐

MIPRYAR LUETUCR comes directly from the patient's specimen and is used to investigate any or all of the microorganisms found at the specimen site

☐☐☐☐☐☐☐☐☐
                12

☐☐☐☐☐☐☐☐☐
3

GOYCALORTIEB the science and study of bacteria

☐☐☐☐☐☐☐☐☐☐☐☐
                 2

OYMOLCYG the science and study of fungi

☐☐☐☐☐☐☐☐
           11

NAORLM AFOLR microorganisms normally found in the body that do not cause disease

☐☐☐☐☐☐☐ ☐☐☐☐☐
      8

RAGA a type of seaweed or algae that helps solidify culture media

☐☐☐☐

CONLOY a group of identical bacteria that grow in a culture from one "parent" bacteria

☐☐☐☐☐☐
      9

OCCCI bacteria that are spherical in form

☐☐☐☐☐
     7

FLGAELAL a whip-like extension that aids in the movement of an organism

☐☐☐☐☐☐☐☐

PITRE DIHS a shallow glass or plastic container that is used to hold a solid culture medium, such as blood agar

☐☐☐☐☐ ☐☐☐☐
      4

LABCILI rod-shaped organisms

☐☐☐☐☐☐☐
6

NOOCLMOASI FOSCINENTI infections people can get from being in a medical setting

☐☐☐☐☐☐☐☐☐☐
              1

☐☐☐☐☐☐☐☐☐☐

☐☐☐☐☐☐☐☐☐☐☐☐
1 2 3 4 5 6 7 8 9 10 11 12

PROCEDURE PRACTICE

Collecting a Sputum Specimen

One of your tasks in the office is to collect sputum specimens. For each step that appears below, write C if the step is correct or I if it is incorrect. If a step is incorrect, briefly describe the correct process.

_____ 1. Gather your equipment and supplies, including the labeled sterile specimen container, gloves, the laboratory request form, and a biohazard transport container.

_____

_____ 2. Wash your hands and put on gloves.

_____

_____ 3. Greet and identify the patient. Explain the procedure. Write the patient's name on the label and place the label inside the container.

_____

_____ 4. Ask the patient to hold his breath.

_____

_____ 5. Ask the patient to expectorate onto a paper towel. Then ask him to move the sample to the specimen container.

_____

_____ 6. Handle the specimen container according to standard precautions. Cap the container right away and put in into a transport container marked *biohazard.* Fill out the proper laboratory requisition slip.

_____

_____ 7. Remove your gloves and wash your hands. Care for and dispose of your equipment and supplies. Clean your work area.

_____

_____ 8. Send the specimen to the laboratory immediately.

_____

_____ 9. Document the procedure.

_____

Matching

Match the microorganism to each of the following examples. The microorganism can have more than one answer.

1. _____ bacteria

2. _____ virus

3. _____ protozoa

4. _____ fungi

5. _____ metazoa

A. athlete's foot

B. rod-shaped bacilli

C. plasmodium

D. candidiasis

E. the agent that causes AIDS

F. spherical shaped cocci

G. tapeworms

H. spirochetes

I. ticks

J. giardia

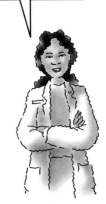

Choose a comfortable environment for studying. For example, if you prefer a quiet environment, try the library.

PRACTICE QUIZ

1. Which of the following is the most effective way to protect yourself in a medical setting?
   a. wash your hands
   b. wear gloves
   c. follow decontamination procedures
   d. use single use disposable equipment

2. Viruses are obligate intracellular parasites. Which of the following statements best describes what that means?
   a. They need a living host to survive and reproduce.
   b. They move from organism to organism via the intracellular fluid.
   c. They produce their own food while living inside another organism.
   d. They are "obligated" to bacteria because they function together to make a person sick.

3. Flatworms belong to the disease-causing group of organisms called:
   a. bacteria.
   b. fungi.
   c. parasites.
   d. viruses.

4. How is spore formation beneficial to a bacillus bacterium?
   a. The spore keeps it from being killed.
   b. The spore produces food for the host.
   c. The spore helps it to move from one organism to another.
   d. The spore makes it harder for the bacteria to be cultured.

5. A bull's-eye shaped rash, headache, fever, and chills are symptoms of:
   a. athlete's foot.
   b. Lyme disease.
   c. malaria.
   d. roundworm infestation.

6. A physician may perform a surgical puncture to obtain a specimen from the:
   a. blood.
   b. skin.
   c. spinal fluid.
   d. sputum.

7. Fungi are opportunistic. What does that mean?
   a. They are not able to spread by contact.
   b. They do not need food or water to survive.
   c. They are much easier to treat or destroy than bacteria.
   d. They are able to cause disease when the chance presents itself.

8. Why do physicians use a tongue depressor when doing a throat culture?
   a. to push the uvula at the back of the throat out of the way
   b. to avoid infecting the tongue with microbes from the throat
   c. to avoid culturing mouth or check microbes in the normal flora
   d. to push the microbes toward the throat so the swab can get them

9. A lab technician observing a bacterium's morphology would be looking at all of the following except:
   a. color.
   b. size.
   c. shape.
   d. metabolic activity.

10. What is the purpose of growing a culture?
    a. to observe how viruses grow and reproduce
    b. to observe how bacteria grow and reproduce
    c. to diagnose and treat a disease based on the type of virus present in the specimen
    d. to diagnose and treat a disease based on the kinds of bacteria present in the specimen

CRITICAL THINKING PRACTICE

Handling Common Specimens

Review the table on the next page and then answer the following questions.

1. You collected a urine specimen at 10:30 A.M. and left it out to be picked up by the lab. At 1:00 P.M., the lab courier still has not arrived. Is the sample still good? Explain.

_____

_____

_____

Handling Common Specimens

Specimen	Collecting	Processing
Urine	Clean-catch midstream with care to avoid contaminating the inside of the container. Don't let stand more than one hour after collection.	Refrigerate if test can't be performed within one hour.
Blood	Handle carefully. Collect in blood culture bottle. Must remain free of contaminants. Requires special preparation of the venipuncture site.	Deliver to lab immediately.
Feces	Collect in clean container. Leave at room temperature if testing for ova (eggs), parasites, or occult blood.	Deliver to lab at once. If delayed, mix with preservative recommended by lab or use transport medium.
Microbiology specimens	Don't contaminate swab or inside of container by touching either to surface other than site of collection. Protect anaerobic specimens from exposure to air.	Transport as soon as possible.

2. The lab is running a test for parasites in feces. After you collected the specimen, you left it at room temperature. It could not be delivered to the lab immediately, so you used a transport medium. Is the sample still good? Explain.

_____

_____

_____

3. You collected blood in a blood culture tube and brought it to the lab immediately after documenting the procedure. Is the sample still good? Explain.

_____

_____

_____

4. You were collecting a microbiology specimen and moving it from a swab to a sterile container. While transferring the specimen, your gloved finger touched the inside of the container. Is the sample still good? Explain.

_____

_____

_____

5. You collected a urine sample at 1:00 P.M. and brought it to the lab for testing. However, the lab was closed for a staff meeting. You brought it back to your work area and placed it in the lab refrigerator. You called the lab at 4:00 P.M. and they said to bring it over. Is the sample still good? Explain.

_____

_____

_____

Preventing Lyme Disease

A 12-year-old patient comes into the office for a physical for summer camp. He will be spending the summer at a wooded camp in the country. His mother is concerned that he will contract Lyme disease. Explain four ways that he can protect himself from Lyme disease.

1. _____

_____

2. _____

_____

3. _____

_____

4. _____

_____

Certification Prep

1. Which bacteria is rod shaped and responsible for tetanus, botulism, and gangrene?
   a. bacilli
   b. spirochete
   c. diplococci
   d. rickettsia

2. What statement best represents the type of infections caused by streptococci?
   a. appendicitis, gastroenteritis
   b. skin infections, colitis
   c. pneumonias, pancreatitis
   d. sore throats, scarlet fever, rheumatic fever

3. Which of the following is NOT an example of a protozoa?
    a. trichomonas
    b. entamoeba
    c. plasmodium
    d. metazoa

4. What is a nosocomial infection?
    a. an infection acquired from a coworker
    b. an infection acquired from a classmate
    c. an infection acquired in a medical setting
    d. an infection acquired from an unknown source or setting

5. What is the purpose of placing antibiotic disks in a culture medium?
    a It is part of the epidemiological study.
    b. It is a method for identifying the microorganism.
    c. It is an important step in research studies.
    d. It tests to see which antibiotic to use in treating the microorganism.

6. Which of the following is NOT an element required for bacterial survival?
    a. oxygen
    b. filtered light
    c. warmth
    d. moisture

7. What is the purpose of a Gram stain?
    a. to differentiate between negative and positive cocci and bacilli
    b. to isolate the Epstein-Barr virus
    c. to identify the number of monocytes and leukocytes
    d. to observe motility of parasites, such as trichomoniasis

8. What is one of the most common infections tested for in a pediatric medical office by a quick test method?
    a. *Bacillus anthracosis*
    b. *Staphylococcus aureus*
    c. *Escherichia coli*
    d. beta-hemolytic streptococcus

9. What should the temperature of an incubator be?
    a. 97–101°F
    b. 35–37°F
    c. 97–101°C
    d. 67–70°F

10. Which of the following personal protective equipment is least necessary when performing tests on microbiology samples?
    a. gloves
    b. goggles or face shield
    c. booties
    d. lab coat or splash-resistant gown

Name _____ Date _____ Time _____

Task: With a partner as the patient, collect a specimen for a throat culture.

Conditions: The student will perform this task under the conditions described in the Procedure Steps, below.

Equipment/Supplies: a tongue blade; a sterile specimen container and swab; gloves; a commercial throat culture kit (for testing in your office); a laboratory request form; a biohazard container (for transport to the lab)

Standards: The student will perform this skill with _____ % accuracy in a total of _____ minutes. *(Your instructor will tell you what the percentage and time limits will be before you begin.)*

Key: 4 = Satisfactory   0 = Unsatisfactory   NA = this step is not counted

Procedure Steps	Self	Partner	Instructor
1. Gather your equipment and supplies, including a tongue blade, a sterile specimen container and swab, gloves, a commercial throat culture kit (for testing in your office), a laboratory request form, and a biohazard container (for transport to the lab).	☐	☐	☐
2. Wash your hands and put on gloves.	☐	☐	☐
3. Greet and identify the patient. Explain the procedure.	☐	☐	☐
4. Ask the patient to sit so a light source is directed at his throat.	☐	☐	☐
5. Remove the sterile swab from its container.	☐	☐	☐
6. Ask the patient to say "ahhh" as you press on the midpoint of the tongue with the tongue depressor. Saying "ahhh" helps reduce the gag reflex.	☐	☐	☐

Continued on back

	Self	Partner	Instructor
7. Now swab the membranes that are suspected to be infected. Normally, you'll touch the side of the throat at the depth of the tissue hanging in the center back of the mouth (uvula). Expose all of the swab's surfaces to the membranes by turning the swab over the membranes. Avoid touching any other areas with the swab.	☐	☐	☐
8. Keep holding the tongue depressor in place while removing the swab from your patient's mouth.	☐	☐	☐
9. Follow the directions on the specimen container for transferring the swab or processing the specimen in the office.	☐	☐	☐
10. Dispose of supplies and equipment in a biohazard waste container. Then, remove your gloves and wash your hands.	☐	☐	☐
11. Route the specimen or store it properly until you can route it.	☐	☐	☐
12. Document the procedure.	☐	☐	☐

Calculation

Total Possible Points: _____

Total Points Earned: _____ Multiplied by 100 = _____ Divided by Total Possible Points = _____ %

Pass   Fail   Comments:

☐   ☐

Student's signature _____ Date _____

Partner's signature _____ Date _____

Instructor's signature _____ Date _____

Name _____ Date _____ Time _____

Task: With a partner as the patient, collect a sputum specimen.

Conditions: The student will perform this task under the conditions described in the Procedure Steps, below.

Equipment/Supplies: a labeled sterile specimen container; gloves; the laboratory request form; a biohazard transport container

Standards: The student will perform this skill with _____ % accuracy in a total of _____ minutes. *(Your instructor will tell you what the percentage and time limits will be before you begin.)*

Key: 4 = Satisfactory   0 = Unsatisfactory   NA = this step is not counted

Procedure Steps	Self	Partner	Instructor
1. Gather your equipment and supplies, including the labeled sterile specimen container, gloves, the laboratory request form, and a biohazard transport container.	☐	☐	☐
2. Wash your hands and put on gloves.	☐	☐	☐
3. Greet and identify the patient. Explain the procedure. Write the patient's name on a label and put the label on the outside of the container.	☐	☐	☐
4. Ask the patient to cough deeply. Tell the patient to use the abdominal muscles to bring secretions up from the lungs.	☐	☐	☐
5. Ask the patient to expectorate directly into the container. Caution him or her not to touch the inside of the container or the specimen will be contaminated. You'll need 5 to 10 mL for most tests.	☐	☐	☐
6. Handle the specimen container according to standard precautions. Cap the container right away and put it into a transport container marked *biohazard*. Fill out the proper laboratory requisition slip.	☐	☐	☐

Continued on back

	Self	Partner	Instructor
7. Care for and dispose of your equipment and supplies. Clean your work area. Then, remove your gloves and wash your hands.	☐	☐	☐
8. Send the specimen to the laboratory immediately.	☐	☐	☐
9. Document the procedure.	☐	☐	☐

Calculation

Total Possible Points: _____

Total Points Earned: _____ Multiplied by 100 = _____ Divided by Total Possible Points = _____ %

Pass   Fail   Comments:

☐   ☐

Student's signature _____ Date _____

Partner's signature _____ Date _____

Instructor's signature _____ Date _____

Hands On **Procedure 7-3:** Collecting a Stool Specimen

Task: With a partner as the patient, explain in detail how to collect a stool specimen, first for ova and parasite testing, then for occult blood testing.

Conditions: The student will perform this task under the conditions described in the Procedure Steps, below.

Equipment/Supplies: a stool specimen container (for ova and parasite testing); an occult blood test kit (for occult blood testing); wooden spatulas or tongue blades

Standards: The student will perform this skill with _____ % accuracy in a total of _____ minutes. *(Your instructor will tell you what the percentage and time limits will be before you begin.)*

Key: 4 = Satisfactory   0 = Unsatisfactory   NA = this step is not counted

Procedure Steps	Self	Partner	Instructor
1. Gather your equipment and supplies, including a stool specimen container (for ova and parasite testing) or occult blood test kit (for occult blood testing) and wooden spatulas or tongue blades. Label the container or test kit with the patient's name.	☐	☐	☐
2. Wash your hands.	☐	☐	☐
3. Greet and identify the patient. Explain the procedure. Also explain any dietary, medication, or other restrictions necessary for the collection. (Don't collect a specimen within four days of a barium procedure.)	☐	☐	☐
4. When collecting a specimen for ova and parasites: • Tell the patient to collect a small amount of the first and last portion of the stool using the wooden spatula and to place the specimen in the container. • Suggest that it's easier if the patient defecates into a disposable plastic container designed to fit on a toilet seat (called a specimen pan, or "top hat") or onto plastic wrap placed over the toilet bowl. • Caution the patient not to contaminate the specimen with urine.	☐	☐	☐

Continued on back

	Self	Partner	Instructor
5. When collecting a specimen for occult blood: • Suggest that the patient obtain the sample from the toilet paper he or she uses to wipe after defecating. Tell the patient to use a wooden spatula to collect the sample. • Tell the patient to smear a small amount of the sample from the spatula onto the slide windows.	☐	☐	☐
6. After the patient returns the stool sample, store the specimen as directed. If you're instructing the patient to take the specimen directly to a laboratory, give the patient a completed laboratory requistion form.	☐	☐	☐
7. Document the date and time of the procedure as well as the instructions that were given to the patient, including the routing procedure.	☐	☐	☐

Calculation

Total Possible Points: _____

Total Points Earned: _____ Multiplied by 100 = _____ Divided by Total Possible Points = _____ %

Pass   Fail   Comments:

☐   ☐

Student's signature _____ Date _____

Partner's signature _____ Date _____

Instructor's signature _____ Date _____

Name _____ Date _____ Time _____

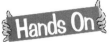 **Procedure 7-4:** Testing a Stool Specimen for Occult Blood

Task: Test a stool specimen for occult blood.

Conditions: The student will perform this task under the conditions described in the Procedure Steps, below.

Equipment/Supplies: gloves; the patient's labeled specimen pack; developer (or reagent drops)

Standards: The student will perform this skill with ____ % accuracy in a total of ____ minutes. *(Your instructor will tell you what the percentage and time limits will be before you begin.)*

Key: 4 = Satisfactory   0 = Unsatisfactory   NA = this step is not counted

Procedure Steps	Self	Partner	Instructor
1. Gather your equipment and supplies, including gloves, the patient's labeled specimen pack, and developer (or reagent drops). Make sure you check the expiration date on the developing solution. You could get inaccurate test results from expired solution.	☐	☐	☐
2. Wash your hands and put on gloves.	☐	☐	☐
3. Open the test window on the back of the pack. Then put a drop of the developer or testing reagent on each window according to the manufacturer's directions.	☐	☐	☐
4. Read the color change within the time specified by the directions. The time is usually 60 seconds.	☐	☐	☐
5. Put a drop of developer (as directed) on the control monitor section or window of the pack. Take note of whether the quality control results are positive or negative, as appropriate.	☐	☐	☐
6. Use proper procedures to dispose of the test pack and gloves. Then, wash your hands.	☐	☐	☐
7. Record the procedure.	☐	☐	☐

Continued on back

Calculation

Total Possible Points: _____

Total Points Earned: _____ Multiplied by 100 = _____ Divided by Total Possible Points = _____ %

Pass   Fail   Comments:

☐   ☐

Student's signature _____ Date _____

Partner's signature _____ Date _____

Instructor's signature _____ Date _____

Name ———————————————————————— Date —————————— Time ——————————

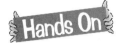 **Procedure 7-5:** Inoculating a Culture Using Dilution Streaking

Task: Inoculate a culture using dilution streaking.

Conditions: The student will perform this task under the conditions described in the Procedure Steps, below.

Equipment/Supplies: the specimen on a swab or loop; gloves; a china marker or permanent lab marker; a sterile or disposable loop; a bacteriological incinerator; a plate

Standards: The student will perform this skill with ____ % accuracy in a total of ____ minutes. *(Your instructor will tell you what the percentage and time limits will be before you begin.)*

Key: 4 = Satisfactory   0 = Unsatisfactory   NA = this step is not counted

Procedure Steps	Self	Partner	Instructor
1. Gather your equipment and supplies, including the specimen on a swab or loop, gloves, a china marker or permanent lab marker, a sterile or disposable loop, a bacteriological incinerator, and a plate.	☐	☐	☐
2. Wash your hands and put on gloves.	☐	☐	☐
3. Label the medium side of the plate with the patient's name, identification number, source of specimen, your initials, and the date. (The patient's name should be on the side of the plate containing the medium because it's always placed upward to keep moisture from dripping onto the culture.)	☐	☐	☐
4. Use your nondominant hand to remove the media side of the plate from its cover. Then turn it over so the media is toward your face.	☐	☐	☐
5. Using a rolling and sliding motion, streak the specimen swab clear across the top quarter of the plate. Start at the top and work your way to the center. If no additional slides or plates are to be set up on this culture, dispose of the swab in a biohazard container. If the inoculating loop is used for lifting microorganisms for a secondary culture, streak in the same way.	☐	☐	☐

Continued on back

	Self	Partner	Instructor
6. If you're inoculating more than one plate using the same sample, perform step 5 on each plate before going on to step 7. Use a new disposable or a sterilized nondisposable loop for each plate.	☐	☐	☐
7. A. Turn the plate a quarter-turn from its previous position. Pass the loop five to six times through the original streaks and down into the new medium approximately a quarter of the surface of the plate. Then make four to five more streaks without entering the originally streaked area. B. If you're inoculating a blood agar plate, you'll perform an additional step at this point to show differentiating hemolytic characteristics of the *Streptococcus* species. Two one-half inch long cuts are made one-fourth inch apart in the middle of the second streaking pattern. To do this, turn the loop sideways and cut half the depth of the loop into the media. With the loop halfway in the media, cut approximately one-fourth to one-half inch long. Repeat this step to make a second cut about one-fourth inch away from the first. Hold the loop at a 45-degree angle so the flap of the media closes off the cut and reduces oxygen growth, which is necessary to show the differentiating hemolytic characteristics of *Streptococcus*.	☐	☐	☐
8. Turn the plate another quarter-turn so that now it's 180 degrees to the original smear. Working in the same way as in step 7A, draw the loop at right angles through the most recently streaked area three to four times. Do not enter the original streaked area this time, however.	☐	☐	☐
9. Care for or dispose of your equipment and supplies properly. Clean your work area. Then, remove your gloves and wash your hands.	☐	☐	☐

Calculation

Total Possible Points: _____

Total Points Earned: _____ Multiplied by 100 = _____ Divided by Total Possible Points = _____ %

Pass   Fail   Comments:

☐   ☐

Student's signature _____ Date _____

Partner's signature _____ Date _____

Instructor's signature _____ Date _____

Name _____ Date _____ Time _____

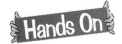 **Procedure 7-6:** Inoculating for Drug Sensitivity Testing (Kirby-Bauer Disk Diffusion Drug Sensitivity) Using "Even Lawn" Streaking

Task: Perform a Kirby-Bauer disk diffusion drug sensitivity test using "even lawn" streaking.

Conditions: The student will perform this task under the conditions described in the Procedure Steps, below.

Equipment/Supplies: a pure broth culture of an organism grown to a standard turbidity (0.5 McFarland standard); gloves; a sterile swab; a china marker or permanent lab marker; a plate

Standards: The student will perform this skill with ____ % accuracy in a total of ____ minutes. *(Your instructor will tell you what the percentage and time limits will be before you begin.)*

Key: 4 = Satisfactory   0 = Unsatisfactory   NA = this step is not counted

Procedure Steps	Self	Partner	Instructor
1. Gather your equipment and supplies, including a pure broth culture of an organism grown to a standard turbidity (0.5 McFarland standard), gloves, a sterile swab, a china marker or permanent lab marker, and a plate.	☐	☐	☐
2. Wash your hands and put on gloves.	☐	☐	☐
3. Label the media side of the plate with the patient's name and/or culture identification number, the source of the specimen, the date, and your initials. Dating a culture helps to distinguish multiple cultures on a patient.	☐	☐	☐
4. Remove the pure culture tube from the test tube rack. Remove the cap from the pure broth culture. A pure culture is necessary to make sure the sensitivity shows a single organism that's causing the infection.	☐	☐	☐

Continued on back

	Self	Partner	Instructor
5. Using your dominant hand, dip the sterile swab into the culture. As you take the swab out of the culture, press and rotate it on the inside of the tube above the level of the broth. This will help remove excess fluid from the swab. Then recap the tube and return it to the rack.	☐	☐	☐
6. Remove the media side of the plate from the cover using your nondominant hand and turn the media toward your face. Remember, the petri dish is always placed on the work surface with the cover down. If you use your nondominant hand for this step, your dominant hand is still free to work with the swab.	☐	☐	☐
7. Starting at one edge of the media, draw the swab down the middle of the plate crossing the diameter of the plate with your streak. Go directly to the next step. Don't change the swab.	☐	☐	☐
8. Using the same swab, streak the plate from side to side at a right angle to the diameter you drew in step 7. Don't leave any space between your streaks in this step. • Use this tip—it's easier to start in the middle of the plate and move toward the top edge. Then rotate the plate 180 degrees and streak the other half of the plate, once again starting in the middle. • If you don't do a good job spreading the bacteria and you leave space between your streaks, it'll be hard to measure the zones of inhibition in a later step. • When you've completed this step, go directly to the next step. Don't change your swab.	☐	☐	☐
9. Now rotate your plate 90 degrees. Streak your plate in the same way you did in step 8. This time, you're streaking parallel to the diameter you drew in step 7. The goal is to spread the bacteria out as much as possible so that when it grows, it will evenly cover every bit of space on the media surface. If you do this step properly, you'll be able to measure the nice round zones of inhibition in a later step.	☐	☐	☐

	Self	Partner	Instructor
10. Rotate your plate 45 degrees and repeat the streaking using the same method as in steps 8 and 9.	☐	☐	☐
11. Within 15 minutes of completing step 10, you must apply the drug disks to the plate using sterile forceps or an automatic dispenser. • Each disk should be pressed down gently using a sterile loop or sterile forceps. Push down until good contact is made with the surface of the agar. • Make sure you pay attention to the time limit on this step. Bacteria reproduce about every 20 minutes. If you wait too long to get the disks on the media, you may get growth where none should exist.	☐	☐	☐
12. Incubate the plates overnight (18 to 24 hours) in an incubator. Incubate with the disk/media side up. The disks won't fall off the media surface when the plate is turned upside down as long as the disks were pressed against the surface of the media.	☐	☐	☐

Calculation

Total Possible Points: _____

Total Points Earned: _____ Multiplied by 100 = _____ Divided by Total Possible Points = _____ %

Pass   Fail   Comments:
☐   ☐

Student's signature _____ Date _____

Partner's signature _____ Date _____

Instructor's signature _____ Date _____

Name _____ Date _____ Time _____

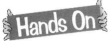 **Procedure 7-7:** Inoculating for Quantitative Culturing or Urine Colony Count Using "Even Lawn" Streaking

Task: Inoculate for quantitative culturing or urine colony count using "even lawn" streaking.

Conditions: The student will perform this task under the conditions described in the Procedure Steps, below.

Equipment/Supplies: a sterile clean-catch urine specimen; a calibrated .01 mL inoculating loop; a china marker or permanent laboratory marker; a plate

Standards: The student will perform this skill with _____ % accuracy in a total of _____ minutes. *(Your instructor will tell you what the percentage and time limits will be before you begin.)*

Key: 4 = Satisfactory   0 = Unsatisfactory   NA = this step is not counted

Procedure Steps	Self	Partner	Instructor
1. Gather your equipment and supplies, including a sterile clean-catch urine specimen, a calibrated .01 mL inoculating loop, a china marker or permanent laboratory marker, and a plate. (Urines are frequently set up on two or three different types of media, for example, blood agar [growth of all organisms], MacConkey [growth of negative rods], or Columbian CAN [growth of positive cocci]. Note the same technique would be used on each plate.)	☐	☐	☐
2. Wash your hands and put on gloves.	☐	☐	☐
3. Label the media side of the plate with the patient's name and/or culture identification number, the source of the specimen, the date, and your initials. Dating the culture helps to distinguish multiple cultures on a patient.	☐	☐	☐
4. Remove the cover from the urine specimen.	☐	☐	☐

Continued on back

	Self	Partner	Instructor
5. Using your dominant hand, dip the calibrated loop into the urine specimen. Hold the loop at a right angle (90 degrees) to the surface of the liquid. Withdraw the loop and make sure there's a film of liquid in the loop. If you can't see a film of liquid, repeat this step.	☐	☐	☐
6. Remove the media side of the plate from the cover using your nondominant hand and turn the media toward your face. Remember, the plate is always placed on the work surface with the cover down. If you use your nondominant hand for this step, your dominant hand is still free to work with the inoculating loop.	☐	☐	☐
7. Hold the loop so the flat side of the loop is parallel to the surface of the media. (This will allow the urine to come off the loop and go onto the plate.) • Starting at one edge of the media, draw the loop down the middle of the plate, crossing the entire diameter of the plate with your streak. • Then go directly to the next step. Don't change loops or sterilize your loop.	☐	☐	☐
8. Using the same loop, now streak the plate from side to side at a right angle to the diameter you drew in step 7. Don't leave any space between your streaks in this step. • Here's a tip. It's easier to start in the middle of the plate and move toward the top edge. Then rotate the plate 180 degrees and streak the other half of the plate, once again starting in the middle. • Then go directly to the next step. Don't change loops or sterilize your loop.	☐	☐	☐
9. Now rotate your plate 90 degrees. Streak your plate in the same way you did in step 8. This time, you're streaking parallel to the diameter you drew in step 7.	☐	☐	☐

	Self	Partner	Instructor
10. Rotate your plate 45 degrees and repeat the streaking using the same method as in steps 8 and 9.	☐	☐	☐
11. Incubate the plate(s) overnight (18 to 24 hours) in an incubator.	☐	☐	☐
12. The visible colonies can be counted the day after incubation and converted to bacteria/mL.	☐	☐	☐

Calculation

Total Possible Points: _____

Total Points Earned: _____ Multiplied by 100 = _____ Divided by Total Possible Points = _____ %

Pass   Fail   Comments:

☐   ☐

Student's signature _____ Date _____

Partner's signature _____ Date _____

Instructor's signature _____ Date _____

Hands On **Procedure 7-8:** Preparing a Wet Mount Slide

Task: Prepare a wet mount slide.

Conditions: The student will perform this task under the conditions described in the Procedure Steps, below.

Equipment/Supplies: the specimen; gloves; a slide, sterile saline or ten-percent potassium hydroxide (KOH); a coverslip; petroleum jelly; a microscope; a pencil or diamond-tipped pen

Standards: The student will perform this skill with _____ % accuracy in a total of _____ minutes. *(Your instructor will tell you what the percentage and time limits will be before you begin.)*

Key: 4 = Satisfactory   0 = Unsatisfactory   NA = this step is not counted

Procedure Steps	Self	Partner	Instructor
1. Gather your equipment and supplies, including the specimen, gloves, a slide, sterile saline or ten-percent potassium hydroxide (KOH), a coverslip, petroleum jelly, a microscope, and a pencil or diamond-tipped pen.	☐	☐	☐
2. Wash your hands and put on gloves.	☐	☐	☐
3. Label the frosted edge of the slide with the patient's name and the date using a pencil or diamond-tipped pen.	☐	☐	☐
4. Put a drop of the specimen on a glass slide with sterile saline or ten-percent potassium hydroxide (KOH).	☐	☐	☐
5. Use a wooden applicator stick to coat the rim of a coverslip with petroleum jelly. • You also can spread a thin layer of petroleum jelly on the heal of your gloved hand, then scrape the edges of the coverslip on it to transfer a thin line to each edge. • Change the glove before the next step if you use this method.	☐	☐	☐

Continued on back

	Self	Partner	Instructor
6. Put the coverslip over the specimen to keep it from evaporating.	☐	☐	☐
7. Examine the slide with a microscope using the 40-power objective lens with diminished light.	☐	☐	☐

Calculation

Total Possible Points: _____

Total Points Earned: _____ Multiplied by 100 = _____ Divided by Total Possible Points = _____ %

Pass   Fail   Comments:

☐   ☐

Student's signature _____ Date _____

Partner's signature _____ Date _____

Instructor's signature _____ Date _____

Hands On Procedure 7-9: Preparing a Dry Smear

Task: Prepare a dry smear.

Conditions: The student will perform this task under the conditions described in the Procedure Steps, below.

Equipment/Supplies: the specimen; gloves; face shield; bacteriological incinerator; slide forceps; slide; sterile swab or inoculating loop; a pencil or diamond-tipped pen

Standards: The student will perform this skill with ＿＿ % accuracy in a total of ＿＿ minutes. *(Your instructor will tell you what the percentage and time limits will be before you begin.)*

Key: 4 = Satisfactory   0 = Unsatisfactory   NA = this step is not counted

Procedure Steps	Self	Partner	Instructor
1. Gather your equipment and supplies, including the specimen, gloves, face shield, bacteriological incinerator, slide forceps, slide, sterile swab or inoculating loop, and a pencil or diamond-tipped pen.	☐	☐	☐
2. Wash your hands and put on gloves.	☐	☐	☐
3. Label the frosted edge of the slide with the patient's name and the date using a pencil or diamond-tipped pen.	☐	☐	☐
4. Hold the ends of the slide by the edges between your thumb and index finger.	☐	☐	☐
5. Spread the specimen on the slide using a swab or inoculating loop and start at the right side of the slide. • Use a rolling motion with the swab or a sweeping motion with the loop. • Spread the material from the specimen gently and evenly over the slide. • The material should thinly fill the center of the slide stopping a half inch from each end. You'll avoid contaminating your gloves this way.	☐	☐	☐

Continued on back

	Self	Partner	Instructor
6. When you're finished placing the specimen on the slide, dispose of the contaminated swab or inoculating loop in a biohazard container. If you're not using a disposable loop, sterilize it using the following steps. • Hold the loop in a bacteriological incinerator for five seconds. Don't use a Bunsen burner for this because it may aerosol your specimen. An incinerator confines any aerosol. • If you'll be reusing the loop, let it cool so that the heat won't kill the bacteria you'll be putting on it. Don't wave the loop in the air. Waving it around can expose it to contamination. Also, don't stab the medium with a hot loop to cool it off because this will create an aerosol.	☐	☐	☐
7. Allow the smear to air dry in a flat position for at least 30 minutes. • Don't wave the slide around in the air or blow on it to speed dry. You could contaminate the specimen with bacteria from your mouth. • Don't apply any heat until the specimen has dried. Heat at this point could damage the microorganisms. • Some specimens, such as Pap smears, must be sprayed with a fixative. (If you spray a fixative, make sure you spray four to six inches above the slide.)	☐	☐	☐
8. Afer drying, hold the dried smear slide with the slide forceps. Then hold the slide in front of the opening of the bacteriological incinerator for eight to ten seconds to "fix" the specimen to the slide. The heat of this process kills the microorganisms and attaches the specimen firmly to the slide.	☐	☐	☐
9. Examine the smear under the microscope or stain it according to your office policy. Usually, the physician will examine the slide to identify the microorganisms in the specimen.	☐	☐	☐

	Self	Partner	Instructor
10. Dispose of equipment and supplies in the correct containers. Remove your gloves and dispose of them as well. Then wash your hands.	☐	☐	☐

Calculation

Total Possible Points: _____

Total Points Earned: _____ Multiplied by 100 = _____ Divided by Total Possible Points = _____ %

Pass   Fail   Comments:

☐   ☐

Student's signature _____ Date _____

Partner's signature _____ Date _____

Instructor's signature _____ Date _____

Hands On Procedure 7-10: Gram Staining a Smear Slide

Task: Gram stain a smear slide.

Conditions: The student will perform this task under the conditions described in the Procedure Steps, below.

Equipment/Supplies: crystal violet stain; a staining rack; Gram iodine solution; a wash bottle with distilled water; alcohol-acetone solution; counterstain (for example, safranin); an absorbent (bibulous) paper pad; a specimen on a glass slide labeled with a diamond-tipped pen or a pencil; immersion oil; a microscope; slide forceps; a stopwatch or timer

Standards: The student will perform this skill with _____ % accuracy in a total of _____ minutes. *(Your instructor will tell you what the percentage and time limits will be before you begin.)*

Key: 4 = Satisfactory 0 = Unsatisfactory NA = this step is not counted

Procedure Steps	Self	Partner	Instructor
1. Gather your equipment and supplies, including crystal violet stain, a staining rack, Gram iodine solution, a wash bottle with distilled water, alcohol-acetone solution, counterstain (for example, safranin), an absorbent (bibulous) paper pad, a specimen on a glass slide labeled with a diamond-tipped pen or a pencil, immersion oil, a microscope, slide forceps, and a stopwatch or timer.	☐	☐	☐
2. Make sure the specimen is heat-fixed to the labeled slide and the slide is at room temperature. See the Hands On procedure on preparing a dry smear for guidance.	☐	☐	☐
3. Wash your hands and put on gloves.	☐	☐	☐
4. Put the slide on the staining rack with the smear side up. The staining rack will collect the dye as it runs off the slide.	☐	☐	☐
5. Flood the smear with crystal violet. Then wait for 30 to 60 seconds.	☐	☐	☐

Continued on back

	Self	Partner	Instructor
6. Hold the slide with slide forceps and tilt it at a 45-degree angle to drain the excess dye. Then rinse the slide with distilled water for about five seconds and drain off the excess water.	☐	☐	☐
7. Put the slide back on the slide rack. Now flood the slide with Gram iodine solution and wait 30 to 60 seconds. The iodine will "fix" the crystal violet to the gram-positive bacteria.	☐	☐	☐
8. Using the slide forceps, hold the slide at a 45-degree angle to drain the iodine solution. While the slide is tilted, rinse the slide with distilled water from the wash bottle for five to ten seconds. Then slowly and gently wash the slide with the alcohol-acetone solution for about five to ten seconds, until no more stain runs off. The alcohol-acetone removes the crystal violet stain from the gram-negative bacteria, but the gram-positive bacteria will keep the purple dye.	☐	☐	☐
9. Immediately rinse the slide with distilled water for five to ten seconds and return it to the rack. The rinsing will stop the decolorizing process.	☐	☐	☐
10. Now, flood the slide with safranin or other appropriate counterstain. Then time a 30- to 60-second wait. The gram-negative bacteria will stain pink or red with the counterstain.	☐	☐	☐
11. Drain the excess counterstain by tilting the slide at a 45-degree angle. After draining the counterstain, rinse the slide with distilled water for five to ten seconds to remove what remains.	☐	☐	☐
12. Gently blot the smear dry with bibulous paper. Be very careful not to disturb the smeared specimen. Wipe off any solution on the back of the slide. You can put the slide between the pages of a bibulous paper pad and press gently to remove any moisture.	☐	☐	☐

	Self	Partner	Instructor
13. Inspect the slide using the oil immersion objective lens. Remember that you are inspecting only for proper preparation. The physician is the one who interprets the slide.	☐	☐	☐
14. Care for or dispose of your equipment and supplies properly. Clean your work area. Remove your gloves and wash your hands.	☐	☐	☐

Calculation

Total Possible Points: _____

Total Points Earned: _____ Multiplied by 100 = _____ Divided by Total Possible Points = _____ %

Pass   Fail   Comments:

☐   ☐

Student's signature _____ Date _____

Partner's signature _____ Date _____

Instructor's signature _____ Date _____

Name _____ Date _____ Time _____

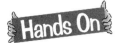 **Procedure 7-11:** Performing Wound Collection Procedure for Microbiological Testing

Task: While role-playing with a classmate, perform wound specimen collection for microbiologic testing, being careful not to contaminate the wound. A classmate will role-play that he or she have an infection on the right calf.

Conditions: The student will perform this task under the conditions described in the Procedure Steps, below.

Equipment/Supplies: soap; water; personal protective equipment; appropriate culturette (verify with physician if culture will be for an aerobic or anaerobic organism)

Standards: The student will perform this skill with _____ % accuracy in a total of _____ minutes. *(Your instructor will tell you what the percentage and time limits will be before you begin.)*

Key: 4 = Satisfactory   0 = Unsatisfactory   NA = this step is not counted

Procedure Steps	Self	Partner	Instructor
1. Verify written order for wound collection in patient's chart.	☐	☐	☐
2. Gather necessary equipment and place patient's name, date, time, and collection site on the appropriate culturette system to be used.	☐	☐	☐
3. Greet patient, verify correct patient, explain procedure, and answer any questions the patient may have.	☐	☐	☐
4. Ask patient to expose affected area. If necessary, leave the room for the patient to disrobe in private. Offer assistance if needed.	☐	☐	☐
5. Assist patient to a supine position and ensure patient is comfortable.	☐	☐	☐
6. Wash hands and put on appropriate personal protective equipment.	☐	☐	☐
7. Open appropriate culturette by peeling back the paper only half-way. This allows the culturette to remain sterile until ready to use.	☐	☐	☐

Continued on back

	Self	Partner	Instructor
8. Assess the wound and determine best area to obtain specimen.	☐	☐	☐
9. Remove culturette with dominant hand. With nondominant hand, open wound site just enough to obtain specimen.	☐	☐	☐
10. Gently place culturette swab in the area of the wound where infection is present and gently twist the swab while in the wound. This ensures sufficient microorganisms have been collected.	☐	☐	☐
11. Place swab of culturette into transport medium and if necessary crush the tip to release the medium. (Verify with instructor which transport system you are using.)	☐	☐	☐
12. Clean area and appropriately dress wound.	☐	☐	☐
13. If necessary, assist patient off table and answer any questions the patient may have.	☐	☐	☐

Calculation

Total Possible Points: _____

Total Points Earned: _____ Multiplied by 100 = _____ Divided by Total Possible Points = _____ %

Pass   Fail   Comments:
☐   ☐

Student's signature _____ Date _____

Partner's signature _____ Date _____

Instructor's signature _____ Date _____